Y0-BVR-966

Clinical Pocket Manual ™

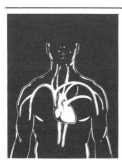

Cardiovascular Care

NURSING86 BOOKS™
SPRINGHOUSE CORPORATION
SPRINGHOUSE, PENNSYLVANIA

Clinical Pocket Manual™ Series

PROGRAM DIRECTOR
Jean Robinson

CLINICAL DIRECTOR
Barbara McVan, RN

ART DIRECTOR
John Hubbard

EDITORIAL MANAGER
Susan R. Williams

EDITORS
Lisa Z. Cohen
Kathy E. Goldberg
Virginia P. Peck

CLINICAL EDITORS
Donna Hilton, RN, CCRN, CEN
Joan E. Mason, RN, EdM
Diane Schweisguth, RN, BSN

COPY SUPERVISOR
David R. Moreau

DESIGNER
Maria Errico

PRODUCTION COORDINATOR
Susan Powell-Mishler

The clinical procedures described and recommended in this publication are based on research and consultation with medical and nursing authorities. To the best of our knowledge, these procedures reflect currently accepted clinical practice; nevertheless, they can't be considered absolute and universal recommendations. For individual application, treatment recommendations must be considered in light of the patient's clinical condition and, before administration of new or infrequently used drugs, in light of latest package-insert information. The authors and the publisher disclaim responsibility for any adverse effects resulting directly or indirectly from the suggested procedures, from any undetected errors, or from the reader's misunderstanding of the text.

Material in this book was adapted from the following series: Nurse's Reference Library, Nursing Photobook, New Nursing Skillbook, Nursing Now, and Nurse's Clinical Library.

Amended reprint, 1986

CPM5-020386

Library of Congress Cataloging-in-Publication Data

Main entry under title:

Cardiovascular care.

(Clinical pocket manual)
"Nursing85 books."
Includes index.
1. Cardiovascular disease nursing—Handbooks, manuals, etc. 2. Cardiovascular system—Diseases—Handbooks, manuals, etc.
I. Springhouse Corporation. II. Series.
RC667.C386 1985   616.1   85-43340
ISBN 0-87434-006-3

CONTENTS

Nursing86 Books™

CLINICAL POCKET MANUAL™ SERIES
Diagnostic Tests
Emergency Care
Fluids and Electrolytes
Signs and Symptoms
Cardiovascular Care
Respiratory Care
Critical Care
Neurologic Care
Surgical Care

NURSING NOW™ SERIES
Shock
Hypertension
Drug Interactions
Cardiac Crises
Respiratory Emergencies
Pain

NURSE'S CLINICAL LIBRARY™
Cardiovascular Disorders
Respiratory Disorders
Endocrine Disorders
Neurologic Disorders
Renal and Urologic Disorders
Gastrointestinal Disorders
Neoplastic Disorders
Immune Disorders

NURSING PHOTOBOOK™ SERIES
Providing Respiratory Care
Managing I.V. Therapy
Dealing with Emergencies
Giving Medications
Assessing Your Patients
Using Monitors
Providing Early Mobility
Giving Cardiac Care
Performing GI Procedures
Implementing Urologic Procedures
Controlling Infection
Ensuring Intensive Care
Coping with Neurologic Disorders
Caring for Surgical Patients
Working with Orthopedic Patients
Nursing Pediatric Patients
Helping Geriatric Patients
Attending Ob/Gyn Patients
Aiding Ambulatory Patients
Carrying Out Special Procedures

NURSE'S REFERENCE LIBRARY®

Diseases	Definitions
Diagnostics	Practices
Drugs	Emergencies
Assessment	Signs and Symptoms
Procedures	

NURSE REVIEW™ SERIES
Cardiac Problems
Respiratory Problems
Gastrointestinal Problems
Neurologic Problems
Vascular Problems

Nursing86 DRUG HANDBOOK™

ASSESSMENT AND
DIAGNOSTIC TESTS

Heart Sounds: Tips for Better Listening Skills

You can sharpen your skills by listening to heart sounds whenever appropriate, performing the technique slowly and precisely in a quiet room. As you work, observe these guidelines:

• Listen to all four auscultatory areas:

—aortic, second right intercostal space

—pulmonic, second left intercostal space

—tricuspid, lower left sternal border

—mitral, cardiac apex.

• To make sure you don't overlook an area, establish a particular order, or sequence, for your auscultation.

• Listen systematically for heart sounds in each area.

• Listen for abnormal heart sounds occurring between the normal heart sounds in each auscultatory area.

Document all your findings and report them to the doctor.

TYPE OF SOUND AND TIMING	LOCATION	POSSIBLE INDICATIONS
Ejection click Onset of systolic ejection	Aortic area, with patient in left lateral position	Aortic stenosis, aortic insufficiency, coarctation of the aorta, aneurysms of the ascending aorta, hypertension with aortic dilation
	Pulmonic area, with patient in left lateral position	Pulmonic stenosis, pulmonary hypertension
Non-ejection click Mid- to late systole	Mitral area, with patient in left lateral position	Prolapsed mitral valve syndrome
Opening snap Early diastole	Fourth intercostal space, at left sternal border	Mitral stenosis
	Second intercostal space, at right sternal border	Tricuspid stenosis

Chest Auscultation: Listening for Heart Sounds

SOUNDS/TIMING	PHYSIOLOGY
S_1 Beginning of systole	• Mitral and tricuspid valves close almost simultaneously, producing a single sound. • S_1 corresponds to the carotid pulse.
Accentuated S_1 Beginning of systole	• Mitral valve is still open wide at the beginning of systole, so the valve slams shut from an open position.
Diminished S_1 Beginning of systole	• Mitral valve has time to float back into an almost closed position before ventricular contraction forces it completely shut, so it closes less forcefully. Softer closure may also be from an immobile, calcified valve.
Split S_1 Beginning of systole	Mitral valve closes slightly before the tricuspid valve.
S_2 End of systole	Pulmonic and aortic valves close almost simultaneously.
Physiologic split S_2 (split on inspiration but not on expiration) End of systole	During inspiration, the pulmonic valve closes later than the aortic valve. (Pulmonic valve closure is normally delayed during inspiration, which causes decreased thoracic pressure and allows more blood into the right heart.)

INDICATION	WHERE TO AUSCULTATE
• Normal	Apex
• During rapid heart rate • Mitral stenosis • After mitral valve disease, such as mitral prolapse	Apex
• First degree heart block • Mitral regurgitation • Severe mitral stenosis with calcified immobile valve	Apex
• Normal in most cases • Right bundle-branch heart block (wide splitting of S_1) • Pulmonary hypertension	Beginning at mitral area and moving toward tricuspid area
• Normal	Aortic and pulmonic areas (base); heard best at aortic area
• Normal: a physiologic S_2 split corresponds to the respiratory cycle.	Aortic and pulmonic areas; heard best at pulmonic area on inspiration

Continued

Chest Auscultation: Listening for Heart Sounds
Continued

SOUNDS/TIMING	PHYSIOLOGY
Persistent wide split S_2 (split on both inspiration and expiration, but more widely split on inspiration) End of systole	Pulmonic valve closes late or (less commonly) the aortic valve closes early.
Fixed split S_2 (equally split on inspiration and expiration) End of systole	Pulmonic valve consistently closes later than aortic valve. Right side of heart is already ejecting a larger volume, so filling cannot be increased during inspiration. The sound remains fixed.
Paradoxical (reversed) S_2 split (widely split on expiration) End of systole	On expiration, aortic valve closes after the pulmonic valve, from delayed or prolonged left ventricular systole. On inspiration, the normal delay of the pulmonic valve closure causes the two sounds to merge.
S_3 (ventricular gallop) Early diastole	Ventricles fill early and rapidly, causing vibrations of the ventricular walls.
S_4 (atrial gallop) Late diastole	Atrium makes an extra effort to fill against increased resistance.

INDICATION	WHERE TO AUSCULTATE
Late pulmonic valve closure: • Complete right bundle-branch heart block, which delays right ventricular contraction. As a result, the pulmonic valve closes later. • Pulmonary stenosis, which prolongs right ventricular ejection	Pulmonic area
• Severe right ventricular failure, which prolongs right ventricular systole • Atrial septal defect, which causes blood return to the right ventricle from lungs, prolonging the ejection	Pulmonic area
• Left bundle-branch heart block (most common cause) • Aortic stenosis • Patent ductus arteriosus • Severe hypertension • Left ventricular failure, disease, or ischemia	Aortic area
• Early congestive heart failure • Ventricular aneurysm • Common in children and young adults	Mitral area and right ventricular area, using stethoscope bell, with patient on his left side
• Hypertensive cardiovascular disease • Chronic coronary artery disease • Aortic stenosis • Hypertrophic cardiomyopathy • Pulmonary artery hypertension	Apex

Characteristics of Heart Murmurs

When timing a murmur, establish if it occurs during diastole or systole. Remember, if you hear a murmur between S_1 and S_2, it's a systolic murmur; between S_2 and the next S_1, a diastolic murmur. Also establish the point in systole or diastole at which the murmur occurs—for example, mid-diastole or late systole.

The intensity of murmurs varies greatly and is graded from I to VI:
• Grade I, very faint

TIMING	QUALITY	PITCH
Systolic ejection	Harsh, rough	Medium to high
Midsystolic	Harsh, rough	Medium to high
	Harsh	High
Holosystolic	Blowing	High
	Blowing	High
Early diastolic	Blowing	High
	Blowing	High
Mid- to late diastolic	Rumbling	Low
	Rumbling	Low

- Grade II, soft and low
- Grade III, prominent but not palpable
- Grade IV, prominent and palpable (you can feel a thrill)
- Grade V, very loud
- Grade VI, audible with the stethoscope off the chest

LOCATION	RADIATION	CONDITION
Pulmonic	Toward left shoulder and neck	Pulmonary stenosis
Aortic and suprasternal notch	Toward carotid arteries or apex	Aortic stenosis
Tricuspid	Precordium	Ventricular septal defect
Mitral, lower left sternal border	Toward left axilla	Mitral insufficiency
Tricuspid	Toward apex	Tricuspid insufficiency
Midleft sternal edge (not aortic area)	Toward sternum	Aortic insufficiency
Pulmonic	Toward sternum	Pulmonary insufficiency
Mitral	Usually none	Mitral stenosis
Tricuspid, lower sternal border	Usually none	Tricuspid stenosis

Assessing Chest Pain

CONDITION	LOCATION AND RADIATION	CHARACTER
Myocardial ischemia (angina pectoris)	• Substernal or retrosternal pain spreading across chest • Radiation possible to inside of either or both arms, the neck, or jaw	• Squeezing, heavy pressure, aching, or burning discomfort
Myocardial infarction	• Substernal or over precordium • Radiation possible throughout chest and arms to jaw	• Crushing, viselike, steady pain
Pericardial chest pain	• Substernal or left of sternum • Radiation possible to neck, arms, back, or epigastrium	• Sharp, intermittent pain (accentuated by swallowing, coughing, deep inspiration, or lying supine)
Pulmonary embolism	• Inferior portion of the pleura • Radiation possible to costal margins or upper abdomen	• Stabbing, knifelike pain (accentuated by respirations)

ONSET AND DURATION	PRECIPITATING EVENTS	ASSOCIATED FINDINGS
• Sudden onset • Usually subsides within 5 minutes	• Mental or physical exertion; intense emotion • Hot, humid weather • Heavy food intake, especially in extreme temperatures or high humidity	• Feeling of uneasiness or impending doom
• Sudden onset • More severe and prolonged than anginal pain	• Occurs spontaneously, with exertion, stress, or at rest	• Dyspnea • Profuse perspiration • Nausea and vomiting • Dizziness, weakness • Feeling of uneasiness or impending doom
• Severe, sudden onset • Usually relieved by bending forward • May occur intermittently over several days	• Upper respiratory tract infection • Myocardial infarction • Rheumatic fever • Pericarditis	• Distended neck veins • Tachycardia • Paradoxical pulse possible with constrictive pericarditis • Pericardial friction rub
• Sudden onset • May last a few days	• Anxiety (associated with coughing)	• Dyspnea; tachypnea • Tachycardia • Cough with hemoptysis

Continued

Assessing Chest Pain
Continued

CONDITION	LOCATION AND RADIATION	CHARACTER
Spontaneous pneumothorax	• Lateral thorax • Does not radiate	• Tearing, pleuritic pain
Infectious or inflammatory processes (pleurisy)	• Pleural • May be widespread or only over affected area	• Moderate, sharp, raw, burning pain
Aortic (dissecting aortic aneurysm)	• Anterior chest • May radiate to thoracic portion of back	• Excruciating, knife-like pain
Esophageal pain	• Substernal • May radiate around chest to shoulders	• Burning, knotlike pain (simulating angina)
Chest wall pain	• Costochondral or sternocostal junctions • Does not radiate	• Aching pain or soreness

ONSET AND DURATION	PRECIPITATING EVENTS	ASSOCIATED FINDINGS
• Sudden onset • Relieved by aspiration of air	• Trauma • Ruptured emphysematous bleb • Anxiety	• Dyspnea; tachypnea • Mediastinal shift • Decreased or absent breath sounds over involved lung
• Occurs on inspiration • Relief usually occurs several days after effective treatment	• Underlying disease of lung, such as pneumonia	• Fever • Cough with sputum production
• Sudden onset • Unrelieved by medication or comfort measures • May last for hours	• Hypertension	• Lower blood pressure in one arm than in other • May have paralysis • May have murmur of aortic insufficiency or pulsus paradoxus • Hypotension and shock
• Sudden onset • Relieved by diet or position change, antacids or belching • Usually brief duration	• May occur spontaneously • Eating	• Regurgitation
• Often begins as dull ache, increasing in intensity over a few days • Usually long lasting	• Chest wall movement	• Symptoms and physical findings vary with specific musculoskeletal disorder

Measuring Cardiac Output

If your patient has a pulmonary artery catheter that's equipped with a thermistor, you can use the thermodilution technique to determine cardiac output. Here's how.

After connecting the catheter's thermistor hub to a special cardiac output computer, inject the indicator solution (usually cold normal saline solution or dextrose 5% in water) into the catheter's proximal lumen. The indicator solution mixes with and cools blood in the heart's right side. When this cooler blood flows past the catheter's distal end, the thermis-

tor detects the temperature drop. The computer than analyzes this information and records the patient's cardiac output on a display screen.

Note: You can't directly measure left-sided cardiac output unless your patient has a catheter in his left ventricle. But because right-sided cardiac output normally equals left-sided output, the value you obtain with the thermodilution technique will reflect left-sided function accurately (except in patients with intracardiac shunts).

Calculating Cardiac Index

To determine at any time if your patient's cardiac output is sufficient for his needs, you'll need to know his cardiac index: cardiac output (expressed in liters/minute) divided by body surface area (in meters squared). To calculate this index, follow these instructions:

First, calculate your patient's body surface area using a nomogram. Find his height and his weight, then use a straightedge ruler to connect these two points. His body surface area is the point where the ruler intersects the center column. For example, if your patient's 70″ (178 cm) tall

and weighs 180 lb (81.6 kg), his body surface area is 2.0 m².

Now you can calculate your patient's cardiac index, using the formula mentioned in the first paragraph.

In the example above, your patient's body surface area is 2.0 m², and let's assume his cardiac output is 6 liters/minute. Therefore, his cardiac index is 3.0 liters/minute/m². Normal cardiac index ranges from 2.5 to 4.2 liters/minute/m², so your patient is within the normal range for his height and weight.

Positioning Chest Electrodes and Marking EKG Strips

To prevent spurious test results, be sure to position chest electrodes as follows:

V_1: fourth intercostal space at right border of sternum
V_2: fourth intercostal space at left border of sternum
V_3: halfway between V_2 and V_4
V_4: fifth intercostal space at midclavicular line
V_5: anterior axillary line (halfway between V_4 and V_6)
V_6: midaxillary line, level with V_4.

Use marking button on the EKG machine to identify chest leads (shown below) and limb leads. Depress button to print a code of long and short dashes (shown below) directly on the EKG strip. (*Note:* Because this code varies, always check the manufacturer's instructions.)

Limb leads		Chest leads	
I:	-	V_1:	— -
II:	--	V_2:	— --
III:	---	V_3:	— ---
aVR:	- —	V_4:	— ----
aVL:	-- —	V_5:	— -----
aVF:	--- —	V_6:	— ------

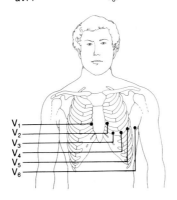

Continuous Cardiac Monitoring

Lead II
Positive (+): left side of chest, lowest palpable rib, midclavicular line
Negative (−): right shoulder, below clavicular hollow
Ground (G): left shoulder, below clavicular hollow

MCL$_1$
Positive (+): right sternal border, lowest palpable rib
Negative (−): left shoulder, below clavicular hollow
Ground (G): right shoulder, below clavicular hollow

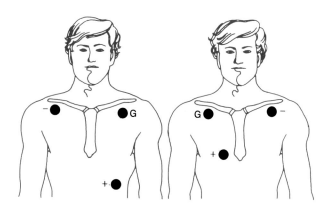

EKG Waveforms: What They Tell Us

You're already familiar with the EKG. As you know, it reflects electrical activity in the heart. But can you interpret each deflection of the EKG waveform?

Electrical stimulation of the heart originates in the sinoatrial (SA) node, which is the heart's sparkplug, or pacemaker. The SA node is located in the upper wall of the right atrium. With regularity, it sends electrical impulses to the atria, stimulating them to contract. The P wave on the EKG waveform appears as the atria depolarize.

Next, the electrical impulse travels to the atrioventricular (AV) junction, where it's slowed. This slowing-down process allows the heart's ventricles to fill with blood from the atria. As this happens, the waveform briefly returns to baseline for the P-R interval. A normal P-R interval lasts approximately 0.12 to 0.2 seconds, and indicates the amount of time it takes an electrical impulse to travel from the SA node through the atria and the atrioventricular junction into the ventricles.

From the AV junction, the impulse travels down the bundle of His, the left and right bundle branches, and the Purkinje fibers.

As the impulse stimulates the ventricles, they contract and eject blood into the pulmonary artery and the aorta. As cells in the ventricles depolarize, the QRS complex appears. Then, the EKG waveform briefly returns to baseline in the S-T segment.

As you can see in the illustration, the Q wave is a negative (downward) deflection; the R wave's a positive (upward) deflection; and the S wave's a negative deflection that follows the R wave. A QRS interval lasts approximately 0.06 to 0.1 seconds. *Note:* Some leads don't display all three waves of the QRS complex.

Continued

EKG Waveforms: What They Tell Us *Continued*

Finally, the cells in the ventricles repolarize, producing a T wave. Occasionally, the T wave's followed by a U wave, indicating repolarization of Purkinje fiber cells. You'll see prominent or inverted U waves if your patient has bradycardia, hypokalemia, or ventricular hypertrophy.

Note: If electrical impulses from the SA node are suppressed or blocked, the AV junction usually takes over and maintains a heart rate of 40 to 60 beats per minute. If the AV junction's impulses are also blocked, ventricular cells initiate electrical conduction. However, the ventricular cells can maintain a heart rate of only 20 to 40 beats per minute.

Dealing With Electrode Placement Problems

Patient is an amputee
• Place the limb lead electrode on his stump.
• If no stump remains, place the limb lead electrode on the trunk near the amputation site.
• Document the unusual electrode placement, and the reason for it.

Patient has severe burns
• Use sterile electrodes.
• Clean the EKG machine carefully before the procedure to minimize the risk of infection.

• If the patient's in reverse isolation, follow the hospital's infection control policy.

Patient has a limb cast
• You may place the electrode under the cast, but make sure it lies flat against his skin.
• Or, place the electrode on skin above cast.
• Document the unusual electrode placement, and the reason for it.

Troubleshooting Cardiac Monitors

PROBLEM/POSSIBLE CAUSES	SOLUTION

Skin excoriation under electrode
- Patient allergic to the electrode adhesive

- Electrode left on skin too long

- Remove electrodes and apply nonallergenic electrodes and non-allergenic tape.

- Remove electrode, clean site, and reapply electrode at new site. *Note:* Do this every 2 or 3 days.

Broken lead wires or a broken cable
- Stress loops not used on lead wires

- Cables and lead wires cleaned with alcohol or acetone, causing brittleness

- Replace lead wires and retape them, using stress loops.

- Clean cable and lead wires with soapy water instead of alcohol or acetone. *Important:* Do not get cable ends wet.

Wandering baseline
- Patient restless

- Chest wall movement during respiration

- Improper application of electrodes; electrode positioned over bone

- Use of nonpolarized electrodes

- Encourage patient to relax.

- Tighten electrode connections.

- Check electrodes and reapply them, if necessary. Place electrodes on fleshy, not bony areas.

- Replace electrodes with polarized ones.

Straight line on monitor (not caused by asystole)
- Improper connection of lead wire to either electrode or cable

- Check cable and electrode connections and adjust them, if necessary.

Continued

ASSESSMENT AND
DIAGNOSTIC TESTS

ASSESSMENT AND
DIAGNOSTIC TESTS

Troubleshooting Cardiac Monitors
Continued

PROBLEM/POSSIBLE CAUSES	SOLUTION

60-cycle interference (fuzzy baseline)

• Electrical interference from other equipment in the room

• Make sure all electrical equipment is attached to a common ground. Check three-pronged plugs to make sure none of the prongs are loose.

• Improper grounding of patient's bed

• Make sure the bed ground is attached to the room's common ground.

Artifact (waveform interference)

• Patient experiencing seizures, chills, or anxiety

• Notify doctor if the patient's having seizures, and treat patient, as ordered. Keep patient warm and reassured. Spend time with him, and discuss his fears.

• Patient restless

• Encourage patient to relax

• Dirty or corroded connections

• Replace dirty or corroded wires.

• Improper application of electrodes

• Check electrodes and reapply them, if needed. Clean the patient's skin well, because skin oils and dead skin cells inhibit conduction.
• Check electrode jelly. If the jelly's dry, apply new electrodes.

• Electrical short circuit in lead wires or cable

• Replace broken equipment. Use stress loops when applying lead wires.

• Electrical interference from other equipment in the room

• Make sure all electrical equipment is attached to a common ground. Check three-pronged plugs to make sure none of the prongs are loose.

Continued

Troubleshooting Cardiac Monitors
Continued

PROBLEM/POSSIBLE CAUSES	SOLUTION

Artifact (waveform interference)
Continued

• Static electricity interference, from decrease in room humidity.

• Regulate room humidity to 40%, if possible.

Double-triggering (P wave and QRS complex, or QRS complex and T wave, are of equal height)
• GAIN setting too high, particularly with MCL$_1$ setting

• Reset GAIN. If possible, monitor patient on MCL$_6$ or another available lead.

Alarm sounds, but you see no evidence of dysrhythmia
• Improper application of electrodes

• Reapply electrodes.

• QRS complex too small to register

• Reset GAIN so that the height of the complex is greater than 1 millivolt.

• QRS complex not registering because of axis shift

• Try monitoring patient on another lead.

• HIGH alarm set too low, or LOW alarm set too high

• Set alarm limits according to patient's heart rate.

• Artifact (waveform interference)

• Check electrodes and reapply them, if necessary.

• Wire or cable failure

• Replace faulty wire or cable.

• Voltage too high or too low

• Adjust GAIN on bedside monitor.

Normal Sinus Rhythm

EKG criteria:
• P wave is normal (of sinus node origin) and upright in lead II.
• P wave precedes each QRS complex.
• PR intervals are normal (0.12 to 0.2 second) and constant.
• RR intervals are constant.
• Heart rate falls between 60 and 100 beats/minute.
Treatment
• None is required.

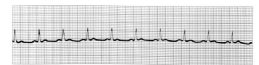

Sinus Tachycardia

EKG criteria:
• Same as normal sinus rhythm except that the heart rate is between 100 and 160 beats/minute.
• P waves are sometimes difficult to see at higher heart rates, but they can usually be found on a 12-lead EKG.
Treatment
• Institute treatment of cause (for example: fever).
• If heart disease has been diagnosed, watch for signs of congestive heart failure. To treat (or prevent) congestive heart failure, give digitalis and diuretics.

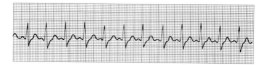

Sinus Bradycardia

EKG criterion:
• Same as normal sinus rhythm but the heart rate is slower than 60 beats/minute (increasing the risk of PVCs). No treatment is needed, except if the condition occurs with hypotension or congestive heart failure.
Treatment
Patients with signs of poor cardiac output or heart failure may require one or more of the following measures:
• Give atropine, 0.4 mg I.V.
• Give I.V. isoproterenol (Isuprel), 0.2 to 1 mg in 250 to 500 ml dextrose 5% in water.
• For low output rates, the doctor will probably insert a temporary pacemaker. For irreversible symptoms of cardiac damage, he'll insert a permanent pacemaker.

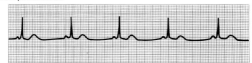

Sinus Arrhythmia

EKG criteria:
• Same as normal sinus rhythm except PP intervals vary slightly.
• PR intervals vary slightly but within normal limits.
• Periods of slow and fast heart rates may alternate, especially in children, depending on crying or respirations.
Treatment
• None. But watch patients with variable PP intervals for premature atrial contractions and other atrial dysrhythmias.

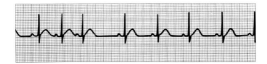

Sinus Arrest (Atrial Standstill)

EKG criteria:
• Same as normal sinus rhythm except that an occasional long pause
follows a regular beat (due to SA node failure to initiate impulse).
• PP interval is normal except that no P wave is seen during pause in
cardiac rhythm.
Treatment
• The pause is not a multiple of the normal PP interval.
• Some patients require no treatment, depending on cause and effect of
sinus arrest.
• If sinus arrest is due to cardiac damage near the SA node, the doctor
will probably insert a temporary pacemaker.
• If SA node is unable to restore normal pacing, a permanent pace-
maker may be needed.

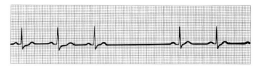

Wandering Pacemaker

EKG criteria:
• P wave changes shape (configuration) and direction because of
changing sites of pacing stimulus.
• PR interval varies from short to normal.
• Variations in rhythm occur because of changes in pacing stimulus.
Treatment
• If acute carditis is present, treat underlying infection.
• If due to digitalis excess, hold dosage for short period.

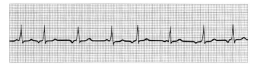

Premature Atrial Contraction (PAC)

EKG criteria:
• Premature P wave may be lost in T wave.
• P wave may have abnormal configuration (flat, slurred, notched, inverted, diphasic, or wide).
• RR interval of premature beat is shorter than normal.
• PR interval may be longer or (occasionally) shorter than normal, depending on location of P wave.
• Pause following PAC is not usually compensatory (that is, the beat following premature beat doesn't occur at normal time because SA node timing was disturbed).
• QRS complex is normal, unless ventricular conduction is delayed or aberrant (follows a different or delayed pathway to ventricles).
Treatment
• Often no treatment is needed.
• If serum potassium is low, give P.O. or I.V. infusion of potassium.
• Give digitalis, as ordered, unless digitalis toxicity is the suspected cause of PACs.
• Give quinidine 200 mg, P.O., usually q.i.d., for patients with organic heart disease.
• Give propranolol if PACs occur in short runs of atrial tachycardia.

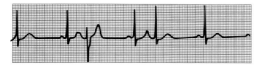

Paroxysmal Atrial Tachycardia (PAT)

EKG criteria:
• Ventricular beats/minute rhythm is perfectly regular with atrial rate of 160 to 250.
• QRS complex is usually narrow.
• P waves may have an abnormal contour or be difficult to see in any of the 12 leads.

Paroxysmal Atrial Tachycardia (PAT) *Continued*

EKG criteria (continued):
• Onset is sudden, often initiated by PAC.
Treatment
• Have patient try Valsalva's maneuver.
• Apply carotid sinus pressure (only doctors do this).
• Give digitalis and verapamil. In some cases, propranolol (Inderal) is also effective.

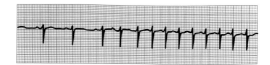

Atrial Flutter

EKG criteria:
• P waves are sawtoothed and referred to as flutter waves (F waves).
• QRS complex is usually narrow.
• Atrial rate is between 250 and 350 beats/minute (usually 300/minute; determine rate by counting number of small squares between points of one sawtooth wave, then dividing into 1,500).
• Varying degrees of AV block (conduction) produce ventricular rates that are ½ to ¼ the atrial rate, giving ratios of 2:1, 3:1, and so forth.
• Ventricular rhythm, although usually regular, can be irregular because conduction ratio varies with each cycle.
• All flutter waves are uniform in width and proceed through QRS complex without interfering with either rhythm.
Treatment
Administer, as ordered, any of the following, either alone or in combination:
• Digitalis (unless flutter is due to digitalis toxicity)
• Propranolol
• Quinidine (after patient is digitalized)

Continued

Atrial Flutter *Continued*

Treatment (Continued):
The doctor may choose either of the following, if necessary:
- Elective cardioversion (if heart rate's greater than 300 beats/minute)
- Temporary atrial pacemaker

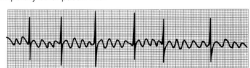

Atrial Fibrillation

EKG criteria:
- Ventricular rhythm is completely irregular, with no pattern to irregularity.
- Atrial fibrillatory (f) waves may be superimposed on T waves.
- Atrial rate (determined as in atrial flutter) is between 350 and 500 beats/minute (could go as high as 700 beats/minute).
- No PR interval is visible.
- QRS complex is usually narrow unless conduction is delayed in ventricles.

Treatment
Administer, as ordered, any of the following, either alone or in combination:
- Digitalis, quinidine, or propranolol to slow ventricular rate and to convert to normal sinus rhythm
- Diuretics for congestive heart failure

The doctor may choose either of the following, if necessary:
- Elective cardioversion
- Temporary pacemaker for low ventricular rates due to AV block

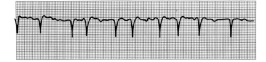

Premature Junctional Contraction (PJC)

EKG criteria:
● RR interval of premature beat is shorter than the patient's normal interval.
● PR interval is short (less than 0.12 second).
● P wave inverts in leads II, III, and aVF, and is upright in aVR and aVL.
● P wave may be before QRS complex, lost in QRS complex, or follow QRS complex and be inverted.
Treatment
● Give potassium supplement if indicated.
● Give digitalis, quinidine, or procainamide if junctional premature beats occur frequently (more than 6/minute).
● If digitalis toxicity is suspected, digitalis should be discontinued.

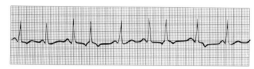

Junctional (Nodal) Tachycardia

EKG criteria:
● Same P wave location and QRS complex as in junctional rhythm.
● Ventricular rate is 60 to 100 beats/minute (slow) or 100 to 220 beats/minute (rapid). (Rapid junctional tachycardia of sudden onset is paroxysmal junctional tachycardia.)
Treatment
● If digitalis toxicity is the cause (likely in paroxysmal junctional tachycardia), withhold dosage and give diuretic to prevent congestive heart failure.
● The doctor may use carotid massage to terminate rapid nodal tachycardia.

Continued

Junctional (Nodal) Tachycardia *Continued*

Treatment (Continued)
- Give propranolol.
- Give phenytoin.
- Give potassium chloride I.V. with I.V. fluids, if ordered.

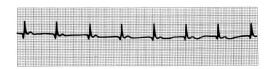

Junctional (Nodal) Rhythm

EKG criteria:
- P wave precedes QRS complex, but PR interval is shorter than 0.11 second. (P wave could be inverted in leads II and III.)
- Or P wave, lost in QRS complex, is not visible.
- Or P wave follows QRS complex and is inverted (retrograde conduction).
- QRS duration is normal unless conduction is aberrant.
- Ventricular rate is between 40 and 60 beats/minute.

Treatment
- If digitalis is suspected as cause, discontinue it.
- Atropine may be indicated.
- Give diuretic to prevent or control congestive heart failure.
- Temporary pacemaker may need to be inserted if cardiac output is poor.

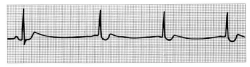

ASSESSMENT AND
DIAGNOSTIC TESTS

First-Degree AV Heart Block

EKG criterion:
• PR interval is prolonged beyond 0.20 second.
Treatment
• In most cases, none.

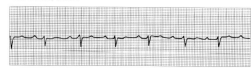

Second-Degree AV Heart Block: Mobitz Type I (Wenckebach)

EKG criteria:
• PR interval becomes longer with each cycle until a P wave lacks a succeeding QRS complex. (Beat drops because of block.)
• RR interval gets progressively shorter (despite prolonged PR interval).
• RR interval containing blocked QRS complex is shorter than intervals of two normal sinus cycles.
• PR interval after the dropped beat is shorter than the one before.
• Blocked beats (dropped QRS complex) are usually cyclic in that a ratio can be established; for example, 3 P waves to 2 QRS complexes = 3:2 ratio (3 impulses, 2 conductions).
Treatment
• Temporary pacemaker may need to be inserted if patient experiences such symptoms as hypotension and/or syncope.

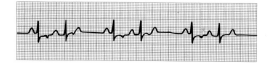

Second-Degree AV Heart Block: Mobitz Type II (4:3 Block)

EKG criteria:
• PR interval is constant.
• QRS complex is periodically dropped after a P wave. (Beat is dropped because of block.)
• QRS complex is wide.
Treatment
• Temporary pacemaker and, eventually, permanent pacemaker may need to be inserted if patient experiences such symptoms as hypotension and/or syncope.

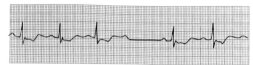

Third-Degree AV Heart Block (Complete Heart Block)

EKG criteria:
• Atrial and ventricular rates differ. Atrial rate is faster than ventricular rate.
• P waves are not related to QRS complexes; they do not indicate ventricular contraction from a sinus beat because impulse is not conducted to ventricles (AV dissociation).
• PR interval varies.
Treatment
• Insertion of permanent pacemaker will probably be necessary.
• Stop digitalis.

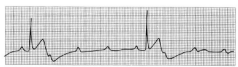

SA Block

EKG criteria:
• Normal sinus rhythm with periodic pauses where an entire cardiac cycle (P, QRS, T) is dropped.
• Dropped cycle doesn't interfere with the normal rhythm; the interval of the dropped beat equals a normal cycle.
Treatment
• Usually none. Determine cause.

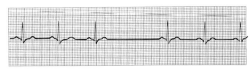

Left Bundle Block

EKG criteria:
• QRS complex is prolonged to 0.12 second or more and is below the isoelectric line in lead V_1.
• Deep S wave appears in V_1.
Treatment
• None may be needed.
• Treat underlying heart disease.

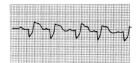

Right Bundle Block

EKG criteria:
• QRS complex is prolonged to 0.12 second or more and is entirely above the isoelectric line in lead V_1.
• Right precordial lead (such as V_1 or V_2) shows RSR' complex with ST depression and inverted T waves.
Treatment
• None may be needed.
• Treat underlying heart disease.

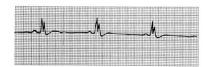

Blocked PAC

EKG criteria:
• P wave occurs early and is often of a different configuration and direction than normal P wave.
• No QRS complex follows premature P wave.
• Interval with dropped QRS is less than a normal cycle.
Treatment
• If numerous blocked PACs occur, consider hypokalemia and check for digitalis or ischemia toxicity.
• Administer digitalis, quinidine, or beta blockers, as ordered.

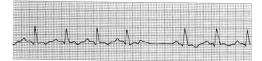

AV Dissociation

EKG criteria:
• QRS complex is normal.
• Atrial rate and ventricular rate are different (no relationship between P waves and QRS complex); ventricular rate is higher.
• PR interval varies or is absent.
Treatment
• If caused by digitalis toxicity, discontinue drug.

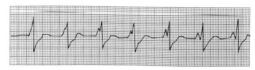

Wolff-Parkinson-White (WPW) Syndrome

EKG criteria:
• PR interval is very short (less than 0.10 second).
• QRS complex is wide (0.11 to 0.14 second) or slurred (looks like bundle branch block).
• Delta waves are present at upstroke of QRS complex.
• Tracing shows runs of paroxysmal tachycardia, which appear as ventricular tachycardia.
Treatment
• Quinidine or procainamide sometimes effective; lidocaine I.V. for wide complex tachycardia.
• Ligation of AV node and permanent bipolar pacemaker.
• Cardioversion.

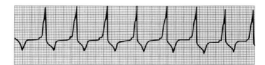

Unifocal and Multifocal PVCs

Note: The following information is the same for both unifocal PVCs and multifocal PVCs.

EKG criteria:
• QRS complex is wide, bizarre, and distorted and usually deflects in opposite direction from patient's normal QRS complex.
• T wave of PVC deflects in opposite direction from QRS complex.
• P waves are not usually visible.
• Compensatory pause follows PVC.

Treatment
These drugs may be administered alone or in combination:
• Lidocaine, 50 to 100 mg, I.V., as a bolus followed by an I.V. of 2 g of lidocaine in 500 ml dextrose 5% in water to be infused at a rate of 1 to 4 mg/minute
• Procainamide (Pronestyl) I.V., 100 mg, I.V. push over 5 to 10 minutes followed by an I.V. of 1 g in 500 ml of dextrose 5% in water at 1 to 4 mg/min.
• Potassium chloride I.V.
• Quinidine by mouth
   Temporary pacemaker may need to be inserted.
   If PVC induced by digitalis, withhold dosage; if induced by hypoxia, give oxygen.
   Note: A malpositioned CVP line, pacing catheter, or pulmonary artery catheter may cause PVCs. Placement should be checked.

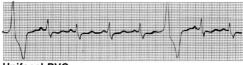

Unifocal PVC

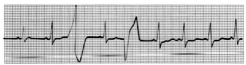

Multifocal PVC

Ventricular Tachycardia

EKG criteria:
• Ventricular rate ranges from 150 to 220 beats/minute.
• QRS complex is wide and bizarre.
• RR intervals usually are regular, but a slight irregularity may occur.
• P waves are obscured by QRS complex.
  Note: A group of three PVCs constitutes a short run of ventricular tachycardia.
Treatment
These drugs may be administered alone or in combination:
• Lidocaine (Xylocaine)
• Procainamide (Pronestyl)
• Quinidine
  Temporary pacemaker may need to be inserted for slow rates with short runs of ventricular tachycardia.
  Direct-current shock may need to be applied if patient is rapidly deteriorating.

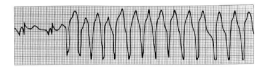

Ventricular Flutter

EKG criteria:
● Rapid, uniform, regular ventricular undulations may exceed 250/minute.
● QRS patterns are not distinct.
Treatment
● Direct-current shock may be applied, followed by lidocaine I.V. and sometimes quinidine or procainamide.
● If first direct-current shock is ineffective, it should be repeated at 6-second intervals.
● Cardiopulmonary resuscitation should be given if direct-current shock fails.

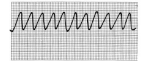

Ventricular Fibrillation

EKG criterion:
● Rapid, chaotic, ventricular rhythm lacks pattern.
Treatment
● Direct-current shock of 200 to 400 W/second should be administered immediately, followed by I.V. lidocaine or procainamide and cardiopulmonary resuscitation.

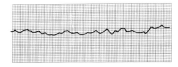

ASSESSMENT AND
DIAGNOSTIC TESTS

Asystole (ventricular)

EKG criteria:
• Either a straight line EKG or some chaotic incomprehensible imprint.
• P wave may be present but no ventricular contraction.
Treatment
• Sharp precordial thump
• CPR (immediate)
• Drugs:
   — Atropine I.V.
   — NaHCO₃ I.V.
   — Intracardiac epinephrine
   — Calcium gluconate I.V.
   — Vasopressors (Levophed, Ar-
amine)
• Temporary pacemaker insertion

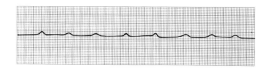

Ashman Phenomenon

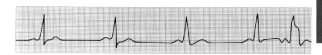

This phenomenon reflects the relationship between the length of the cardiac cycle and refractoriness of cardiac tissue. Theoretically, an aberration of conduction will occur when a short cycle follows a long one, because the refractory period varies with the length of the cycle. Any impulse that ends a short cycle that is preceded by a long one is more likely to encounter refractory tissue. For example, in sinus bradycardia complicated by premature atrial contraction (PAC), the cycle of sinus bradycardia is long; but because PAC shortens the cardiac cycle, the PAC will be conducted aberrantly, usually in an RBB pattern.

In the past, the Ashman phenomenon was associated with atrial fibrillation. However, because so much concealed conduction occurs in atrial fibrillation, it's not possible to tell exactly when bundle branch activation, one of the mechanisms of aberrant conduction, occurs.

Points to Remember About Dysrhythmias

• Dysrhythmias are becoming more common, possibly because improved monitoring techniques are detecting them more often.

• Dysrhythmias are generally classified according to their site or origin (ventricular or supraventricular). Ventricular dysrhythmias are potentially more life-threatening than supraventricular dysrhythmias.

• You need to monitor the patient for factors which predispose him to dysrhythmia, such as fluid and electrolyte imbalance and signs of drug toxicity, especially with digoxin.

• After recognizing dysrhythmia, you must accurately assess the patient's cardiac, electrolyte, and overall clinical status, noting especially whether the dysrhythmia is life-treatening

• When treating a dysrhythmia, you must evaluate the patient's cardiac output. Consider potentially progressive or ominous dysrhythmias in determining your course of action. Administer medications as ordered, and prepare to assist with medical procedures, if indicated.

• To prevent dysrhythmia in a post-operative cardiac patient, you must provide adequate oxygen and reduce the heart's workload while carefully maintaining metabolic, neurologic, respiratory, and hemodynamic status.

• New advances in the treatment and detection of dysrhythmias—new antiarrhythmic drugs, cardiac pacemakers, electrical cardioversion, cardiopulmonary resuscitation, and endocardial stripping (for ventricular dysrhythmias)—offer a brighter outlook.

• Dysrhythmias that contribute to sudden death may occur due to coronary artery spasm, especially with unstable angina, aortic stenosis, cardiomyopathy, pulmonary hypertension, dissecting or ruptured aortic aneurysm, massive intracerebral and subarachnoid hemorrhage, massive gastrointestinal hemorrhage, aspiration of a food bolus.

Characteristic EKGs in MI

Infarctions in different sites of the heart cause EKG changes. Recognizing these significant changes will help you assess your patient.

• An *inferior wall myocardial infarction (MI)* will show typical pattern changes—a pathologic Q wave, S-T segment elevation, and T wave inversion—in leads II, III, and aVF.

• Sometimes an inferior or posterior wall infarction will involve the lateral wall as well. *Lateral wall involvement* will cause a reduced R wave, a T wave inversion, and, in some cases, an elevation of the S-T segment in the lateral leads I, V_5, V_6, and aVL.

• A *posterior wall infarction* causes a tall R wave and upright T wave in V_1.

• An *anterior myocardial infarction* will produce a typical infarction pattern in leads I, aVL, and V_2 to V_6.

• An *anteroseptal infarction* will cause the typical pattern in leads V_1 to V_4.

• An *anterolateral infarction* will produce the typical pattern in leads I, V_5, and V_6.

• An infarction within the anterolateral surface of the left ventricle—a *high anterolateral infarction*—will produce typical changes in leads I, aVL, and V_6.

Change for the better

These EKG patterns gradually return to normal. Recovery after a myocardial infarction can be divided into four phases:

PHASE I (acute phase): Immediately after onset or within 48 hours, leads reflecting the injured area show abnormal Q waves, an elevated S-T segment, and inverted T waves. Reciprocal changes, such as S-T depression, occur in leads reflecting the uninjured area.

PHASE II: This phase covers the gradual return of the elevated S-T segment to the baseline.

PHASE III: Most T waves return to normal or near-normal configuration.

PHASE IV (stabilized phase): An abnormal Q wave may be the only sign of infarction.

These four phases may be complete in 3 days or may take up to 10 days to complete. Remember always to interpret EKGs in light of other laboratory findings, such as cardiac enzymes (creatinine phosphokinase, lactic dehydrogenase, serum glutamic-oxaloacetic transaminase), and the patient's symptoms.

His Bundle Electrography

In this schematic view, a multipolar electrode catheter is inserted
through the superior vena cava, right atrium, and tricuspid valve. When
the catheter is withdrawn, the tip moves downward along the ventricle
wall, and as it passes the His bundle—located in the septum—a characteristic spike appears on the electrogram.

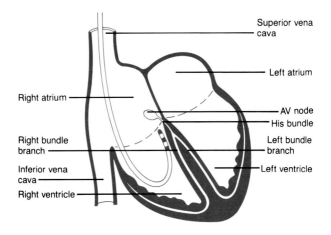

Adapted with permission from Mark E.
Josephson and Stuart F. Seides,
Clinical Cardiac Electrophysiology:
Techniques and Interpretations
(Philadelphia: Lea & Febiger, 1979).

Complications of Cardiac Catheterization

Cardiac catheterization imposes more patient risk than most other diagnostic tests. Although the incidence of such complications is low, they are potentially life-threatening and require careful observation during the procedure.

Keep in mind that some complications are common to *both* left heart and right heart catheterization; others result only from catheterization of one side. In either case, complications require that you notify the doctor and carefully document the complication and its treatment.

LEFT OR RIGHT HEART CATHETERIZATION

COMPLICATION	SIGNS AND SYMPTOMS	NURSING CONSIDERATIONS
Myocardial infarction *Possible causes:* • Emotional stress induced by procedure • Blood clot dislodged by catheter tip travels to a coronary artery (left heart catheterization only)	• Chest pain, possibly radiating to left arm, back, and/or jaw • Cardiac dysrhythmias • Diaphoresis, restlessness, and/or anxiety • Thready pulse • Fever • Peripheral cyanosis, causing cool skin	• Keep resuscitation equipment available. • Give oxygen or other drugs, as ordered. • Monitor patient continuously, as ordered.
Dysrhythmias *Possible cause:* • Cardiac tissue irritated by catheter	• Irregular heartbeat • Irregular apical pulse • Palpitations	• Monitor patient continuously, as ordered. • Administer antiarrhythmic drugs, if ordered.

Continued

Complications of Cardiac Catheterization
Continued

LEFT OR RIGHT HEART CATHETERIZATION

COMPLICATION	SIGNS AND SYMPTOMS	NURSING CONSIDERATIONS
Cardiac tamponade *Possible cause:* • Perforation of heart wall by catheter	• Dysrhythmias • Increased heart rate • Decreased blood pressure • Chest pain • Diaphoresis • Distant heart sounds	• Give oxygen, if ordered. • Prepare patient for emergency surgery, if ordered. • Monitor patient continuously, as ordered.
Infection (systemic) *Possible causes:* • Poor aseptic technique • Catheter contaminated during manufacture, storage, or use	• Fever • Increased pulse rate • Chills and tremors • Unstable blood pressure	• Collect urine, sputum, and blood samples for culture, as ordered. • Monitor vital signs.
Hypovolemia *Possible causes:* • Diuresis from angiography contrast medium	• Increased urinary output • Hypotension	• Replace fluids by giving patient 1 to 2 glasses of water every hour, or maintain I.V. at a rate of 150 to 200 ml/hr, as ordered. • Monitor fluid intake and output closely. • Monitor vital signs.

Continued

Complications of Cardiac Catheterization
Continued

LEFT OR RIGHT HEART CATHETERIZATION

COMPLICATION	SIGNS AND SYMPTOMS	NURSING CONSIDERATIONS
Pulmonary edema *Possible cause:* • Excessive fluid administration	• Early stage: tachycardia, tachypnea, dependent rales, diastolic (S_3) gallop • Acute stage: dyspnea; rapid, noisy respirations; cough with frothy, blood-tinged sputum; cyanosis with cold, clammy skin; tachycardia; hypertension	• Administer oxygen and give medications, as ordered. • Restrict fluids and insert a Foley catheter, as ordered. • Monitor the patient continuously, as ordered. • Maintain the patient's airway, and keep him in semi-Fowler's position. • Apply rotating tourniquets, as ordered. • Keep resuscitation equipment available.
Hematoma or blood loss at insertion site *Possible cause:* • Bleeding at insertion site from vein or artery damage	• Bloody dressing • Limb swelling • Decreased blood pressure • Increased heart rate	• Elevate limb, and apply direct manual pressure. • When the bleeding's stopped, apply a pressure bandage. • If bleeding continues, or if vital signs are unstable, notify doctor.

Continued

ASSESSMENT AND
DIAGNOSTIC TESTS

Complications of Cardiac Catheterization
Continued

LEFT OR RIGHT HEART CATHETERIZATION

COMPLICATION	SIGNS AND SYMPTOMS	NURSING CONSIDERATIONS
Reaction to contrast medium *Possible cause:* • Allergy to iodine	• Fever • Agitation • Hives • Itching • Decreased urinary output, indicating kidney failure	• Administer antihistamines to relieve itching, as ordered. • Administer diuretics to treat kidney failure, as ordered. • Monitor fluid intake and output closely.
Infection at insertion site *Possible cause:* • Poor aseptic technique	• Swelling, warmth, redness, and soreness at site • Purulent discharge at site	• Obtain drainage sample for culture. • Clean site, and apply antimicrobial ointment, if ordered. Cover site with sterile gauze pad. • Review and improve aseptic technique.
LEFT HEART CATHETERIZATION **Arterial embolus or thrombus in limb** *Possible causes:* • Injury to artery during catheter insertion, causing blood clot	• Slow or faint pulse distal to insertion site	• Notify doctor. He may perform an arteriotomy and Fogarty

Continued

Complications of Cardiac Catheterization
Continued

LEFT HEART CATHETERIZATION

COMPLICATION	SIGNS AND SYMPTOMS	NURSING CONSIDERATIONS
Arterial embolus or thrombus in limb *Continued* • Plaque dislodged from artery wall by catheter	• Loss of warmth, sensation, and color in arm or leg distal to insertion side	catheterization to remove embolus or thrombus. • Protect affected arm or leg from pressure. Keep it at room temperature, and maintain it at a level or slightly dependent position. • Administer a vasodilator, to relieve painful vasospasm, if ordered.
Cerebrovascular accident (CVA) *Possible cause:* • Blood clot or plaque dislodged by catheter tip travels to brain	• Hemiplegia • Aphasia • Lethargy • Confusion or decreased level of consciousness	• Monitor vital signs closely. • Keep suctioning equipment nearby. • Administer oxygen, as ordered.

RIGHT HEART CATHETERIZATION
Thrombophlebitis
Possible cause:

• Vein damaged during catheter insertion	• Vein is hard, sore, cordlike, and warm. Vein may look like a	• Elevate arm or leg and apply warm, wet compresses.

Continued

Complications of Cardiac Catheterization
Continued

RIGHT HEART CATHETERIZATION

COMPLICATION	SIGNS AND SYMPTOMS	NURSING CONSIDERATIONS
Thrombophlebitis *Continued*	red line above catheter insertion site. • Swelling at site	• Administer anticoagulant or fibrinolytic drugs, if ordered.
Pulmonary emboli *Possible cause:* • Blood clot or plaque dislodged by catheter tip travels to lungs	• Shortness of breath	• Place patient in high Fowler's position. • Administer oxygen, if ordered.
Vagal response *Possible cause:* • Vagus nerve endings irritated in SA node, atrial muscle tissue, or AV junction	• Hypotension • Decreased heart rate	• Administer atropine, if ordered. • Keep patient supine.

Cardiac Pressures in Recumbent Adults

CHAMBER OR VESSEL	PRESSURE (mm Hg)*
Right atrium	6 (mean)
Right ventricle	30/6**
Pulmonary artery	30/12** (mean, 18)
Left atrium	12 (mean)
Left ventricle	140/12**
Pulmonary artery wedge	±1 to 2 mm Hg to LA pressure

*Upper limits **Peak systolic and end-diastolic

Adapted with permission from H. Kasparian, et al., "Interpreting Cardiac Catheterization Data," *Postgraduate Medicine* 57,4:67, April 1975.

Clarifying Hemodynamic Concepts

Understanding the following hemodynamic concepts (afterload, cardiac output, ejection fraction, preload, stroke volume) will help you assess and manage your cardiac patient's condition more effectively.

Afterload
• The tension in the ventricular muscle during contraction. The amount of force needed to overcome pressure in the aorta determines afterload in the left ventricle. Afterload is also known as *intraventricular systolic pressure.* (In the right ventricle, *afterload* may be used to describe the amount of force needed to overcome pressure in the pulmonary artery.)

Cardiac output
• Probably the most important circulatory measurement of left ventricular function. It describes the volume of blood ejected by the left ventricle in a given period, usually 1 minute. Normal cardiac output ranges from 4 to 8 liters/minute. Cardiac output may also refer to blood ejected by the right ventricle.

(You can calculate this for either ventricle by multiplying stroke volume times heart rate.)

Ejection fraction
• The ratio of the amount of blood expelled from each ventricle in one contraction (systolic volume) to the ventricle's total capacity (end-diastolic volume). A healthy heart at rest has an ejection fraction of 60% to 70%. The 30% to 40% reserve contributes to the next stroke volume.

Preload
• The force exerted on the ventricular muscle at end-diastole that determines the degree of muscle fiber stretch. Preload is a key factor in the heart's contractility—the more cardiac muscles are stretched during diastole, the more powerfully they contract in systole. Preload is also known as *ventricular end-diastolic pressure.*

Stroke volume
• The output of each ventricle in one contraction, normally 60 to 70 ml/beat. Stroke volume is also known as *systolic volume.*

Choosing an Arterial Catheter Site

ADVANTAGES	DISADVANTAGES

Brachial artery

ADVANTAGES	DISADVANTAGES
• Larger than radial artery and easily located. • Site readily observed and maintained. • Bleeding can usually be prevented or controlled by direct pressure. • Pressure readings may be more accurate than those taken from the radial artery, since the site's closer to the heart.	• Risk of damage to median nerves during catheter insertion. • Risk of tissue damage if artery occludes, because patient will lack adequate collateral circulation to the lower arm. • Patient's elbow must be splinted to stabilize the catheter, causing joint stiffness. • Thrombosis may occur if artery's small or if patient has low cardiac output.

Radial artery

ADVANTAGES	DISADVANTAGES
• Easily located. • Ulnar artery provides good collateral circulation to hand. • Site readily observed and maintained. • Anatomically stable; radius acts as natural splint.	• Small lumen in vessel; catheter insertion may be difficult and painful. • Pressure readings may be inaccurately high, because site is so far from heart.

Femoral artery

ADVANTAGES	DISADVANTAGES
• Large lumen in vessel; may be the easiest artery to locate and puncture in an emergency. • Anatomically stable; femur acts as natural splint.	• Risk of damage to nearby femoral vein and major nerves. • High risk of thrombosis. • Risk of tissue damage if artery occludes, because of limited collateral circulation. • Difficult to secure catheter. • Difficult to bandage insertion site and keep it clean. • Difficult to prevent and control bleeding.

Continued

Choosing an Arterial Catheter Site
Continued

ADVANTAGES	DISADVANTAGES

Dorsalis pedis artery

• May be used if other sites are unavailable because of burns or other injures.	• High risk of thrombosis. • Produces false high blood pressure readings, because site is so far from heart.

Preparing Your Patient for Insertion of an Arterial Catheter

If your patient needs an arterial line, make sure you've prepared him properly before the doctor begins the insertion. Here's how:

• Explain the procedure to your patient. Tell him that the doctor will give him a local anesthetic to minimize discomfort. Then, take time to answer his questions completely. Remember, catheter insertion is easier if your patient's relaxed.

• Find out if your patient's allergic to the povidone-iodine skin prep or the local anesthetic. If he's allergic to either, tell the doctor.

• If the doctor's chosen the radial artery for the insertion site, check your patient's ulnar and radial artery circulation using the Allen's test.

• Document your patient's pulse distal to the chosen insertion site. If his pulse weakens later while the arterial catheter's in place, suspect inadequate blood circulation.

• Position your patient so he's comfortable. Make sure the insertion site's level and easily accessible.

• Protect your patient's bed linens by placing a bedsaver pad under the insertion site. Cover the bedsaver pad with a sterile towel.

How the Pulmonary Artery Catheter Works

The doctor inserts the balloon-tipped, multilumen PA catheter into the patient's internal jugular or subclavian vein (or, in some cases, into the basilar vein of the antecubital fossa). After the catheter's inserted, the doctor advances it into the right atrium. There, he inflates the balloon to help propel the catheter through the right ventricle and into the pulmonary artery. Inflated, the balloon lodges in a pulmonary capillary, allowing pulmonary capillary wedge pressure (PCWP) measurement through the opening at the tip. Deflated, it rests in the pulmonary artery, allowing diastolic and systolic PA pressure readings.

What do readings from a catheter that never enters the left heart have to do with measuring left-heart pressure? The balloon blocks blood flow from the right atrium and ventricle, so the only pressure the catheter tip senses is from areas around the balloon. During diastole, when the aortic valve is closed but the mitral valve is open, the pressure the tip senses reflects that of the left ventricle: PCWP approximately equals LVEDP (left ventricular end-diastolic pressure).

Four-Lumen Pulmonary Artery Catheter

Pulmonary artery catheters are made of pliable, radiopaque polyvinylchloride. The illustration on page 51 shows a 110 cm (about 43¼″) catheter, marked in 10-cm increments. It has distal and proximal lumens, which are fluid-filled for pressure monitoring; a thermistor lumen, which holds the wires connecting the thermistor to the cardiac output computer; and a balloon inflation lumen with valve. As a result, this catheter can measure several pressures, as well as cardiac output.

Since catheters vary depending on their manufacturer, consult the manufacturer's manual for additional details.

Continued

Four-Lumen Pulmonary Artery Catheter
Continued

Thermistor hub:
Connects to the cardiac output computer to measure cardiac output.

Distal lumen hub:
Attaches to pressure line to measure pulmonary artery pressure and pulmonary artery wedge pressure. I.V. flush solution exits from the distal port.

Balloon inflation valve:
Receives the proper amount of gas (air or carbon dioxide) to inflate the balloon.

Proximal lumen hub:
Attaches to pressure line to measure right atrial central venous pressure. To measure cardiac output, disconnect from pressure line and inject solution. I.V. flush solution or injectate solution exits from proximal port.

Distal lumen port:
Rests in the pulmonary artery.

Thermistor:
Detects blood temperature changes used to measure cardiac output. Located about 1½" (3.8 cm) from the catheter tip.

Balloon:
Expands around catheter, when inflated, without occluding distal port.

Proximal lumen port:
Rests in the right atrium.

Pulmonary Artery Catheter Insertion

As the catheter is directed through the right heart chambers to its wedge position, it produces distinctive waveforms that are important indicators of the catheter's position in the heart on the oscilloscope screen.

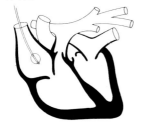

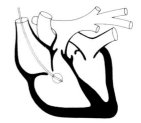

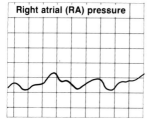

Right atrial (RA) pressure

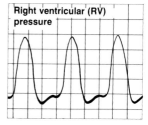

Right ventricular (RV) pressure

1. When the catheter tip reaches the right atrium from the superior vena cava, the waveform on the oscilloscope screen or readout strip looks like this. When it does, the doctor inflates the catheter's balloon, which floats the tip through the tricuspid valve into the right ventricle.

2. When the catheter tip reaches the right ventricle, the waveform looks like this.

Continued

Pulmonary Artery Catheter Insertion
Continued

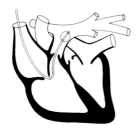 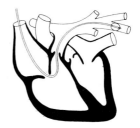

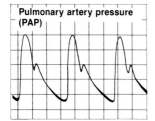

3. A waveform like this one indicates that the balloon has floated the catheter tip through the pulmonic valve into the pulmonary artery. A dicrotic notch should be visible in the waveform, indicating the closing of the pulmonic valve.

4. Blood flow in the pulmonary artery then carries the catheter balloon into one of the pulmonary artery's many smaller branches. When the vessel becomes too narrow for the balloon to pass through, the balloon wedges in the vessel, occluding it. The monitor then displays a pulmonary capillary wedge pressure (PCWP) waveform like this one.

Troubleshooting Hemodynamic Pressure Monitoring

PROBLEM/POSSIBLE CAUSES	SOLUTIONS
No waveform • Power supply turned off • Monitor screen pressure range set too low • Loose connection in line • Transducer not connected to amplifier • Stopcock off to patient • Catheter occluded or out of blood vessel	• Check power supply. • Raise monitor screen pressure range, if necessary. Rebalance and recalibrate equipment. • Tighten loose connections. • Check and tighten connection. • Position stopcock correctly. • Use fast-flush valve to flush line. • Try to aspirate blood from catheter. If the line still won't flush, notify the doctor and prepare to replace the line.
Drifting waveforms • Improper warm-up • Electrical cable kinked or compressed • Temperature change in room air or I.V. flush solution	• Allow monitor and transducer to warm up for 10 to 15 minutes. • Place monitor's cable where it can't be stepped on or compressed. • Routinely zero and calibrate equipment 30 minutes after setting it up. This allows I.V. fluid to warm to room temperature.
Line fails to flush • Stopcocks positioned incorrectly • Inadequate pressure from pressure bag	• Make sure stopcocks are positioned correctly. • Make sure pressure bag guage reads 300 mm Hg.

Continued

Troubleshooting Hemodynamic Pressure Monitoring
Continued

PROBLEM/POSSIBLE CAUSES	SOLUTIONS

Line fails to flush
Continued
● Kink in pressure tubing or blood clot in catheter

● Check pressure tubing for kinks.

● Try to aspirate the clot with a syringe.
● If the line still won't flush, notify the doctor and prepare to replace the line, if necessary. *Important:* Never use a syringe to *flush* a hemodynamic line.

Artifact (waveform interference)
● Patient movement

● Electrical interference

● Catheter fling (tip of pulmonary artery catheter moving rapidly in large blood vessel or heart chamber)

● Wait until the patient is quiet before taking a reading.
● Make sure electrical equipment is connected and grounded correctly.
● Notify the doctor. He may try to reposition the catheter.

Falsely high readings
● Transducer balancing port positioned below patient's right atrium
● Flush solution flow rate too fast

● Air in system

● Catheter fling (tip of pulmonary artery catheter moving rapidly in large blood vessel or heart chamber)

● Position balancing port level with the patient's right atrium.
● Check flush solution flow rate. Maintain it at 3 to 4 ml/hour.
● Remove air from the lines and the transducer.
● Notify the doctor. He may try to reposition the catheter.

Continued

Troubleshooting Hemodynamic Pressure Monitoring
Continued

PROBLEM/POSSIBLE CAUSES	SOLUTIONS
Falsely low readings	
• Transducer balancing port positioned above right atrium	• Position balancing port level with the patient's right atrium.
• Transducer imbalance	• Make sure the transducer's flow system isn't kinked or occluded, and rebalance and recalibrate the equipment.
• Loose connection	• Tighten loose connections.
Damped waveform	
• Air bubbles	• Secure all connections.
	• Remove air from lines and transducer.
	• Check for and replace cracked equipment.
• Blood clot in catheter or stopcock	• Refer to "Line fails to flush" on page 55.
• Blood flashback in line	• Make sure stopcock positions are correct.
	• Tighten loose connections and replace cracked equipment.
	• Flush line with fast-flush valve.
• Transducer line	• Replace the transducer dome if blood backs up into it.
	• Make sure the transducer is kept at the level of the right

Continued

Troubleshooting Hemodynamic Pressure Monitoring
Continued

PROBLEM/POSSIBLE CAUSES	SOLUTIONS

Damped waveform
Continued

atrium at all times. Improper levels give false high or low pressure readings.

• Transducer position
  • Reposition if the catheter is against vessel wall.

• Transducer not balanced properly
  • Check transducer cable for occlusion or compression.
  • Level the transducer's balancing port with the patient's right atrium, and balance the transducer to atmospheric pressure.
  • Recalibrate the monitor with the transducer.

• Arterial catheter out of blood vessel or pressed against vessel wall
  • Try to aspirate blood to confirm proper placement in the vessel. If you can't aspirate blood, notify the doctor and prepare to replace the line. *Note:* Bloody drainage at the insertion site may indicate catheter displacement. Notify the doctor immediately.

• Pulmonary artery (PA) catheter pressed or wedged against blood vessel wall
  • Deflate balloon on PA catheter completely.
  • Ask patient to cough. This may jolt the catheter free.
  • Fast flush the catheter, using the fast flush valve. This also may jolt it free.
  • Notify the doctor, so he can reposition the catheter, if necessary.
  • Prepare the patient for a chest X-ray to confirm correct catheter placement.

How to Measure CVP

No matter which type of catheter your patient has in place, you can monitor his central venous pressure (CVP) in two ways: either with a transducer and monitor, or with a fluid-filled manometer. If your patient has a PA catheter in place, connect the PA catheter's *proximal lumen hub* to the transducer or to the manometer.

Unlike the transducer and monitor, which measure CVP (mm Hg), a manometer measures CVP (cm H_2O). If the doctor changes your patient's monitoring setup from a transducer and monitor to a manometer (or vice versa), you'll need to know how to convert the measurements. Otherwise, you'll be unable to tell if your patient's CVP changes significantly. Keep these formulas in a handy place:

- To convert cm H_2O to mm Hg: cm $H_2O \div 1.36 =$ mm Hg
- To convert mm Hg to cm H_2O: mm Hg $\times 1.36 =$ cm H_2O.

How to Use a Manometer

To take a CVP reading with a manometer, clamp the manometer to an I.V. pole so it is vertical. Then, hang the I.V. and prime the tubing. Hang the I.V. 30″ to 36″ above the insertion site.

Attach a stopcock to the manometer's tubing. Then, connect the I.V. tubing to the open side of the stopcock

Turn the stopcock to I.V.-TO-MANOMETER position. Fill the manometer column with I.V. solution until it's almost full. (Don't fill it to the top, or you'll contaminate the manometer's air filter.)

Now, turn the stopcock to I.V.-TO-PATIENT position, and flush the tubing. When the air's expelled, close the flow clamp. Now, the doctor will connect the patient's CVP catheter to this tubing.

Open the flow clamp and adjust the I.V. flow rate, as ordered.

To take a CVP reading, position the patient flat. Lower the manometer and line up the *zero mark* on the manometer scale with the patient's right atrium.

Turn the stopcock to MANOMETER-TO-PATIENT position. The fluid will drop in the manometer column, stopping when the pressure equals that of the patient's CVP.

Expect the fluid column to rise and fall slightly as the patient breathes. Note the highest level the fluid reaches, and take your reading from the base of the meniscus.

The Risks of PA Catheterization

POTENTIAL PROBLEMS	NURSING CONSIDERATIONS
Dysrhythmias—from the catheter knotting, from irritation of the endocardium or heart valves, or from migration into the right ventricle	• Examine the catheter before insertion to be sure it's free of kinks. • Keep the catheter taped securely to the insertion site. • Monitor the patient's EKG closely, especially during insertion. • Keep equipment and drugs available for dysrhythmia treatment.
Air embolism—from a balloon rupture	• Test the balloon before catheter insertion. • Inflate the balloon gradually and only to recommended levels. • If you feel no resistance, stop the inflation and notify the doctor.
Pulmonary embolism—from a blood clot migrating from the catheter tip	• Maintain continuous heparinized flush to minimize clot formation. • If you suspect clot formation, don't flush the catheter. Instead, try to aspirate the clot. If you're unsuccessful, notify the doctor.

Continued

The Risks of PA Catheterization
Continued

POTENTIAL PROBLEMS	NURSING CONSIDERATIONS
Sepsis—from poor aseptic technique during insertion or from irritation or contamination of the insertion site	• Maintain strict aseptic technique. • Change the insertion site dressing, tubing, and stopcocks every 24 hours or according to hospital policy. • Keep the doctor aware of how long the catheter's been in place. He'll try to keep catheterization at any one site under 72 hours. • Observe for signs of infection. Notify the doctor if infection develops, and culture the insertion site, catheter tip, and blood, as ordered.
Endocarditis—from poor aseptic technique or from vascular or endocardial injury	• Maintain strict aseptic technique. • Minimize catheter manipulation. • Observe for signs of infection. Notify the doctor if infection develops.
Pneumothorax—from lung laceration or injection of air into the pleural space during insertion. (Most common with subclavian insertion.)	• During insertion, keep the patient in Trendelenburg's position. For a subclavian insertion, place a rolled towel between his shoulders.

Continued

ASSESSMENT AND DIAGNOSTIC TESTS

The Risks of PA Catheterization
Continued

POTENTIAL PROBLEMS	NURSING CONSIDERATIONS
Pneumothorax *Continued*	• Instruct the patient to stay as still as possible during insertion. If he's restless, the doctor may order sedation. • Before infusing large volumes of fluid, be sure the doctor checks the patient's lung expansion and catheter placement.
Pulmonary infarction of PA perforation—from prolonged or frequent wedging or from migration of the catheter into a PA branch. *Note:* Thrombosis is another possible cause; see guidelines for pulmonary embolism, on page 59.	• Inflate the balloon to recommended levels. • Deflate the balloon as soon as you get a PCWP reading. If the PA waveform doesn't appear, check to see that the balloon has deflated. Also, try positioning the patient on either side to dislodge the catheter. If this fails, notify the doctor at once. • Keep the catheter taped securely to the insertion site.
Bleeding at the insertion site—from vessel injury or catheter movement	• Keep the catheter taped securely to the insertion site. • Minimize the patient's movement. • If direct pressure doesn't halt the bleeding, notify the doctor.

All About Congenital Heart Defects

Are you aware that about 8 out of every 1,000 children are born with heart defects? And among premature infants, the incidence increases two to three times or more, depending on birth weight. So as a pediatric nurse, you need to know the basics about these serious disorders.

Sometimes, congenital heart defects are difficult to diagnose because they don't appear until weeks, months, or even years after birth. Minor congenital heart defects are particularly difficult to diagnose because of vague, transient, or self-limiting symptoms. Defects may become more recognizable as greater demands are placed on the heart.

Generally, heart defects are classified into two groups: cyanotic and acyanotic. Here's how they differ.

As you know, the heart's powerful left side normally produces significantly higher pressure than its right side. A cyanotic defect alters this situation, causing abnormally high pressure in the heart's *right* side. This condition, combined with other abnormalities associated with some defects, may permit shunting of unoxygenated blood from the heart's right side to its left side. The subsequent flow of unoxygenated blood from the left ventricle to the body causes cyanosis.

Acyanotic defects, on the other hand, don't produce these abnormal pressure changes. So, a septal defect, for example, permits shunting of oxygenated blood from the heart's high-pressure *left* side to its low-pressure *right* side. Because the left ventricle still ejects oxygenated blood to the body, no cyanosis results. But keep in mind that an acyanotic defect may *become* cyanotic if its effects worsen.

Clearly, either type of defect may threaten your patient's health—and even his life. Your skill at recognizing early signs and symptoms is crucial. Read the chart on the next page to learn more about common congenital heart defects.

Guide to Congenital Heart Defects

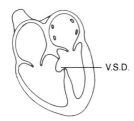

V.S.D.

VENTRICULAR SEPTAL DE-
FECT (V.S.D.)

Abnormal opening in the ventricular septum, allowing
blood to shunt between the
left and right ventricles. Most
common congenital heart disorder; occurs more often in
premature than in full-term infants.

Characteristics
- Causes oxygenated blood
from left ventricle to mix with
unoxygenated blood in right
ventricle (left-to-right shunt)
- Acyanotic, unless very large
or coupled with other disorder
causing right-to-left shunt
- Usually asymptomatic at
birth; becomes evident after
2 weeks

- May improve or close spontaneously approximately 6
months after birth
- If opening fails to close 1 to
2 years after birth, may
cause pulmonary valve ob-
struction
- May act as life-saving
safety valve when coupled
with other severe heart defects, such as transposition of
the great vessels
- If opening's large, may result in cardiac complications,
such as congestive heart failure and bacterial endocarditis
- Large VSD may eventually
cause pulmonary vascular
disease and pulmonary artery
hypertension

Signs and symptoms
- Overactive precordium, especially after feeding
- Within 6 weeks after birth,
harsh systolic murmur heard
best in third and fourth left intercostal spaces; associated
with palpable thrill; murmur
may be only sign of disorder
- Increased right ventricular
and pulmonary artery pressure
- If condition's severe: poor

Continued

Guide to Congenital Heart Defects
Continued

VENTRICULAR SEPTAL DEFECT (V.S.D.)
Continued

growth; labored breathing; and pattern of frequent feeding

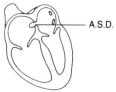

A.S.D.

ATRIAL SEPTAL DEFECT (A.S.D.)

Opening or gap between the left and right atria, allowing left-to-right shunting of blood between chambers. Condition caused by delayed or improper closure of foramen ovale cordis or atrial septal wall. More common in females. Classified into three types: ostium secundum, located in the fossa ovalis cordis (most common); sinus venosus, located in upper atrial septum; and ostium primum, located in lower atrial septum.

Characteristics
• May go unrecognized because of sign subtlety
• May cause atrial dysrhythmias, secondary to right atrial overload
• May interfere with conduction system
• May cause pulmonary hypertension, if defect is severe
• May act as a life-saving safety valve if associated with a severe heart defect, such as Tetralogy of Fallot
• May cause complications, such as pulmonary embolism; bronchopulmonary infections; and pulmonary artery rupture
• May close spontaneously within 1 year after birth

Signs and symptoms
• Soft, pulmonic midsystolic murmur heard at second or third left intercostal space
• In infants, dyspnea on exertion, fatigue, orthopnea
• In older children with a large defect, frail, left precordial bulge.

Continued

Guide to Congenital Heart Defects
Continued

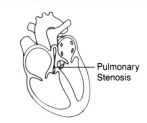

Pulmonary
Stenosis

PULMONARY STENOSIS

Narrowing of pulmonic valve,
usually resulting from altered
or distorted pulmonary valve
cusps or right ventricular outflow obstruction. Classified
into three types: valvular,
subvalvular, and supravalvu-
lar.

Characteristics
• Usually acyanotic and
asymptomatic, unless defect's
severe
• Associated with a history of
maternal rubella
• Causes increased right
ventricular pressure to overcome obstruction; this, in
turn, elevates right atrial pres-

sure, leading to increased
systemic venous blood pressure
• May result in right ventricular failure
• Low or normal pulmonary
artery pressure

Signs and symptoms
• Dyspnea
• Fatigue
• Extremity coldness, peripheral cyanosis
• Subjective complaints (such
as tiring easily) that increase
with age
• Precordial pain possible
• In valvular pulmonary stenosis, systolic ejection murmur associated with a thrill
(best heard at upper left sternal border); if defect's severe,
murmur may radiate over precordium and back
• If right ventricular end-diastolic pressure increases,
right ventricle hypertrophy occurs
• To relieve respiratory distress, child may assume
squatting position

Continued

Guide to Congenital Heart Defects
Continued

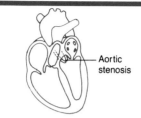

Aortic stenosis

AORTIC VALVULAR STENOSIS

Narrowing of aortic valve or left ventricular outflow obstruction. More common in males.

Characteristics
• Acyanotic, unless defect's severe
• Usually asymptomatic in infants and children
• Severe obstruction causes increased left ventricle pressure to maintain aortic pressure; this condition may lead to left ventricle hypertrophy

Signs and symptoms
• In infants, atypical systolic murmur and possible intractable congestive heart failure
• Systolic ejection click followed by systolic ejection murmur and a thrill felt at the second right intercostal space or suprasternal notch
• Irritability
• Tachycardia
• Dyspnea and fatigue on exertion
• Angina pectoris
• Syncope
• Pale skin
• Narrow pulse pressure
• Weak peripheral pulses
• Possible abdominal pain
• Diaphoresis
• Epistaxis

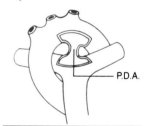

P.D.A.

PATENT DUCTUS ARTERIOSUS (P.D.A.)

Patent duct between the descending aorta and pulmonary artery bifurcation, allowing shunting from the
Continued

Guide to Congenital Heart Defects
Continued

PATENT DUCTUS ARTERIO-SUS (P.D.A.) *Continued*

pulmonary artery to the aorta. Normally, ductus arteriosus closes shortly after birth. More common in females.

Characteristics
• Associated with history of prematurity, first trimester maternal rubella, coxsackievirus infection, or birth at high altitude
• Acyanotic; usually asymptomatic
• May be accompanied by coarctation of aorta
• May cause pulmonary congestion, especially in premature infants
• May lead to complications, such as congestive heart failure, ductus arteriosus aneurysm (causing blood to dissect between duct walls), spontaneous aneurysm rupture, and recurrent respiratory infections

Signs and symptoms
• Continuous murmur with characteristic machinelike quality, loudest at second and third left intercostal spaces; murmur may obscure S_2 heart sound and be only sign of disorder
• Dyspnea on exertion
• Precordial asymmetry; in infants, overactive precordium
• Widened pulse pressure
• Full or bounding pulses
• Pulmonary artery hypertension with right-to-left shunt, and right atrial and ventricular hypertrophy

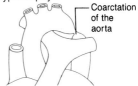

Coarctation of the aorta

COARCTATION OF THE AORTA

Constriction of the aorta. More common in males. Classified into two types: preductal and postductal. Defect may occur anywhere on aortic arch.

Characteristics
• Acyanotic
• Symptoms usually occur in

Continued

Guide to Congenital Heart Defects
Continued

COARCTATION OF THE AORTA
Continued

either early infancy or adult-hood (20 to 30 years old)
• Collateral circulation may develop around defect, mini-mizing pressure changes
• If condition's severe, may lead to complications, such as congestive heart failure.
• Frequently associated with bicuspid aortic valve
Signs and symptoms
• Elevated blood pressure and bounding pulses proximal to defect, hypotension, and weak or absent pulses distal to defect
• Dizziness
• Fainting
• Headache
• Epistaxis
• Cold feet
• Systolic ejection click heard at base and apex of heart; associated with systolic or continuous murmur between scapulae
• Pulmonary hypertension
• Aneurysm proximal to de-fect

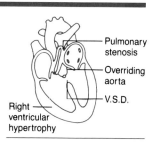

Pulmonary stenosis
Overriding aorta
V.S.D.
Right ventricular hypertrophy

TETRALOGY OF FALLOT

Combination of four defects: ventricular septal defect (V.S.D.), overriding aorta, pul-monary stenosis, and right ventricular hypertrophy
Characteristics
• Unoxygenated blood is shunted through V.S.D.
• Oxygenated and unoxygen-ated blood are mixed in left ventricle and pumped out aorta, causing cyanosis
• Pulmonary stenosis re-stricts blood flow to lungs and increases right ventricular pressure
• Defects may cause compli-cations such as iron defi-ciency anemia, polycythemia, coagulation disorders,

Continued

Guide to Congenital Heart Defects
Continued

TETRALOGY OF FALLOT
Continued

paradoxical embolism, cerebral infarction, and abscesses

Signs and symptoms
- Cyanosis
- Loud systolic ejection murmur heard along left sternal border; may diminish or obscure pulmonic S_2 component
- Finger and toe clubbing
- Dyspnea
- On palpation, possible cardiac thrill at left sternal border
- In neonate: intense cyanosis after patent ductus arteriosus closes, severe dyspnea on exertion, syncope, limpness, and occasional convulsions; if defect is untreated, it may be fatal
- To compensate for respiratory distress, child may assume characteristic squatting position
- Respiratory distress and fatigue during feeding
- Growth retardation

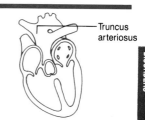

Truncus arteriosus

TRUNCUS ARTERIOSUS

Failure of embryonic arterial trunk to separate into aorta and pulmonary artery. Resulting single vessel overrides ventricles and carries blood for both pulmonary and systemic circulation.

Characteristics
- Ventricular septal defect (V.S.D.) always present
- Common trunk may have 2 to 6 valve cusps
- Usually fatal within 6 months if untreated

Signs and symptoms
- Cyanosis
- Systolic murmur about 1 month after birth
- Fatigue
- Dyspnea
- Failure to thrive

Continued

Guide to Congenital Heart Defects
Continued

CARDIOVASCULAR DISORDERS

TRUNCUS ARTERIOSUS
Continued

- Parasternal lift
- Loud decrescendo diastolic murmur possible
- Ejection click
- S_2 has only one component because of single valve in common trunk
- Tachypnea
- Rales
- Recurrent respiratory infections
- Wide pulse pressure possible
- Congestive heart failure, usually indicating rapid physical decline
- Hepatomegaly possible

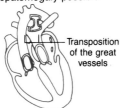

Transposition of the great vessels

TRANSPOSITION OF GREAT VESSELS

Aorta leaves right ventricle; pulmonary artery leaves left ventricle. Usually associated with ventricular septal defect (V.S.D.), atrial septal defect (A.S.D.), and/or patent ductus arteriosus (P.D.A.). More common in males.

Characteristics
- Associated with history of maternal diabetes
- Causes unoxygenated blood to flow through right atrium and ventricle and out aorta to systemic circulation; oxygenated blood flows from lungs to left atrium and ventricle and out pulmonary artery to lungs
- May be fatal unless V.S.D., A.S.D., or P.D.A. develops as safety valve for two independent circulations

Signs and symptoms
- Cyanosis
- High birth weight possible
- Signs of congestive heart failure within 12 to 24 hours after birth
- Poor sucking reflex
- Systolic murmur, if V.S.D. is present
- Hepatomegaly
- Metabolic acidosis

Angina Pectoris

Chief complaint
• *Chest pain:* may be dull or burning, or described as pressure, tightness, heaviness; builds and fades gradually; may be in abdomen; may radiate to jaw, teeth, face, or left arm
• *Dyspnea:* possible, with sense of constriction around larynx or upper trachea
• *Fatigue:* absent
• *Irregular heartbeat:* may be present; patient complains of palpitations or skipped beats
Peripheral changes: none

History
• Risk factors include family history of coronary artery disease, arteriosclerotic heart disease, cerebrovascular accident, diabetes, gout, hypertension, renal disease, obesity caused by excessive carbohydrate and saturated fat intake, smoking, lack of exercise, stress (Type A personality)
• Higher incidence in men over age 40; lower incidence in women prior to menopause
• Precipitating factors include exertion, stress, cold or hot weather, and emotional excitement

Physical examination
• Inspection usually reveals patient anxiety; skin may be quite pale, cool, and damp
• Palpation reveals tachycardia
• Auscultation reveals change in blood pressure, especially during anginal attack; transient rales associated with congestive heart failure; paradoxical splitting of S_2 possible; an atrial gallop may be present if the patient is in the left lateral position; S_3, suggesting a temporary decompensation of the left ventricle, may occur; S_3 and S_4 sounds may form a summation gallop.

Diagnostic studies
• Electrocardiogram may show depressed ST segments during ischemia attack but may be within normal limits; atrioventricular conduction defect
• Thallium stress imaging or stress electrocardiogram may show ischemic area
• Nitroglycerin test may be used to differentiate angina pain from myocardial infarction; with angina, 0.4 mg of nitroglycerin administered at the onset of chest pain will relieve the pain rapidly.
• Coronary arteriogram may show narrowing of coronary vessels.

Always Ask the Patient:

• *Is the pain better or worse when you breathe in or out?* Anginal pain isn't affected by respiration.
• *Is the pain better or worse when you change your body positions?* Again anginal pain usually isn't affected by position changes.
• *Does the pain seem deep or superficial; mild or intense?* Cardiac pain seems deep and unusually intense; noncardiac pain is typically described as mild "soreness" or dull aching.
• *Can you point to the pain with one finger?* Cardiac pain tends to be diffuse, not sharply localized.

Diagnostic Profile for Angina

EKG abnormalities during and after exercise
• Chest X-rays
• Cardiac catheterization before surgery
• Nitroglycerin will shorten an attack of anginal pain or increase the tolerance to exercise
Stable angina: occurs over a long time in same pattern of onset, duration, and intensity of symptoms
Unstable angina: frequency, intensity, and duration of symptoms increase as atherosclerotic process progresses; about 50% of patients will infarct within 3 to 18 months after onset
Prinzmetal's angina: chest discomfort at rest due to coronary artery spasm causes transient S-T segment elevation and pain
Angina decubitus: chest discomfort that occurs in the recumbent position, relieved by sitting or standing
Nocturnal angina: occurs only at night, but not necessarily in the recumbent position
Intractable angina: chronic chest discomfort that is physically incapacitating and refractory to medical treatment

Acute Myocardial Infarction

Chief complaint
• *Chest pain:* sudden, but not instantaneous, onset of constricting, crushing, heavy weightlike chest pain occurring at any time—not relieved by nitroglycerin; located centrally and substernally; may build rapidly or in waves to maximum intensity in a few minutes; may be accompanied by nausea and vomiting
• *Dyspnea:* present; may be accompanied by orthopnea, cough, and wheezing
• *Fatigue:* present; indicated by weakness and apprehension
• *Irregular heartbeat:* may be present; patient complains of palpitations or skipped beats
• *Peripheral changes:* peripheral cyanosis, with decreased perfusion

History
• Risk factors same as in angina pectoris
• Past medical history may include episodes of angina pectoris

Physical examination
• Fever after 24 hours
• Inspection reveals anxiety, tenseness, sense of impending doom, nausea, vomiting, and possibly distended neck veins, sweating, pallor, cyanosis, and shock
• Palpation reveals tachycardia or bradycardia and weak pulse
• Auscultation reveals normal or decreased blood pressure (less than 80 mm Hg), significant murmurs that may preexist or occur with ruptured septum or ruptured papillary muscle, diminished gallop rhythm, pericardial friction rub and rales
• In severe attack: shock, decreased urinary output, pulmonary edema

Diagnostic studies
• EKG at onset shows elevated ST segment, which then returns to baseline; T waves become symmetrically inverted; abnormal Q waves present; may also show dysrhythmias
• White blood cell count shows leukocytosis on second day (lasts 1 week); rises on second or third day
• Enzyme testing shows elevated CPK and CPK-MB (in muscle and brain) initially; then increased SGOT

How A.M.I. Affects Mechanisms of Heart Function

CARDIOVASCULAR DISORDERS

Contractility. Reduction in coronary blood flow may reduce myocardial contractility and pumping efficiency. If the reduction is severe or total, myocardial tissue may not contract at all.

Besides losing contractility, myocardial tissue thins as necrosis progresses. The stresses of normal heart operation may cause this thinned, noncontractile tissue to bulge or rupture. If poor contractility is widespread, overall left ventricular function decreases, lowering stroke volume and cardiac output while raising end-diastolic volume and pressure.

Severe pump failure can occur when loss of contractility affects 40% or more of the myocardium.

Compliance. Myocardial ischemia affects the intake side of pumping operations and output. Decreased compliance impairs ventricular filling and increases the heart's work load creating more oxygen demand. If the rise in demand isn't met, the infarct may enlarge.

Excitability. Depolarization and repolarization depend on an exchange of sodium and potassium ions across myocardial cell membranes. The sodium-potassium pump that accomplishes this exchange runs on energy created by the breakdown of adenosine triphosphate (ATP) to adenosine diphosphate (ADP). Because an ischemic myocardium lacks sufficient oxygen, it reverts to anaerobic metabolism. The lactic acid produced by anaerobic metabolism causes a pH-level drop that depresses the sodium-potassium pump, altering electrical activity. Ischemia also causes an increase in intracellular sodium and a decrease in intracellular potassium, changing the threshold potentials for depolarization and repolarization.

Altered excitability can lead to dysrhythmias, from which hypotension, shock, and death may follow in minutes.

Infarction Sites and Structural Injury

INFARCTION SITES	BLOCKED ARTERY	INJURED STRUCTURES
Anteroseptal, anterior	Left anterior descending (LAD)	• Anterior wall of left ventricle • Anterior interventricular septum • Apex of left ventricle • Bundle of His and bundle branches • Papillary muscles
Anterolateral, posterior, lateral	Left circumflex (LC)	• Left atrium • Lateral and posterior left ventricle • Posterior interventricular septum • Sinoatrial (SA) node* • Atrioventricular (AV) node*
Inferior/posterior	Right coronary (RC)*	• Right atrium (occasionally) • Right ventricle (occasionally) • Inferior left ventricle • SA node* • AV node* • Posterior and inferior interventricular septum

CARDIOVASCULAR DISORDERS

*Damage to these structures varies from one individual to the next, depending on anatomic differences. In about 9 out of 10 persons, the RC artery supplies the AV node; in those remaining, the LC artery supplies the AV node. The RC artery also supplies the SA node in over half of all persons; in the rest, the LC artery performs this function.

Normal Cardiac Serum Enzyme Levels

CARDIAC ENZYME	NORMAL SERUM LEVELS
Creatine phosphokinase (CPK)	Male: 23 to 99 units/liter Female: 15 to 57 units/liter
Serum glutamic-oxaloacetic transaminase (SGOT)	8 to 20 units/liter
Lactic dehydrogenase (LDH)	48 to 115 units/liter
Alpha-hydroxybutyric dehydrogenase (HBD)	114 to 290 units/ml
Serum glutamic-pyruvic transaminase (SGPT)	Male: 10 to 32 units/liter Female: 9 to 24 units/liter

Implications of Elevated Cardiac Enzymes

CPK
- myocardial infarction
- alcohol intoxication
- diabetes mellitus
- skeletal muscle trauma
- intramuscular injections
- vigorous exercise
- convulsions

- pulmonary embolism
- surgery

SGOT
- liver disease
- skeletal muscle disease
- intramuscular injection
- shock

Continued

ELEVATION (POST MI)

ONSET	PEAK	END
Within 1 day	Within 1 day	1 to 2 days
1 day	1 to 2 days	4 to 6 days
2 days	2 to 5 days	4 to 6 days
2 days	3 days	14 days

SGPT levels usually remain near normal except in patients with liver disease.

Implications of Elevated Cardiac Enzymes
Continued

SGOT
Continued
- congestive heart failure with passive hepatic congestion
- prolonged tachycardia
- pericarditis
- hemolysis
- pulmonary embolism or infarction

LDH
- anemia
- leukemia
- liver disease
- hepatic congestion
- renal disease
- neoplasm
- pulmonary embolism or infarction
- myocarditis
- skeletal muscle disease
- intramuscular injection
- hemolysis
- shock

How Serum Enzyme Levels Change in Myocardial Infarction

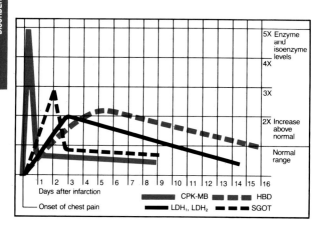

Cardiac Enzymes: Critical Clues

Patients suspected of having a myocardial infarction (MI) always need serial EKGs and serial enzyme studies. Enzymes are catalytic proteins that vary in concentration, depending on the tissue in which they appear. Since a damaged tissue releases enzymes into the blood, enzyme studies tell what organ is damaged and to what extent. *(Note:* Because testing methods vary from hospital to hospital, be sure to check your hospital's lab manual for normal values.)

Draw blood samples for an enzyme study very carefully, since a traumatic venipuncture can falsely elevate results. For example, red blood cells that contain LDH, HBD, and SGOT can release these enzymes in cases of hemolysis. Look for three highly specific enzymes to help diagnose an MI:

SGOT—serum glutamic-oxaloacetic transaminase, an enzyme found mainly in the heart muscle and the liver and to some degree in skeletal muscle, kidney, and red blood cells.

LDH—lactic dehydrogenase, found in the heart, liver, kidney, brain, skeletal muscle, and erythrocytes. Since it's found in tissues outside the heart, laboratories separate LDH into five subgroups called isoenzymes. The LDH_1 and LDH_2 isoenzymes are the myocardial fraction that rises after MI. An LDH_2 value higher than LDH_1 is indicative of myocardial damage. Some laboratories routinely measure hydroxybutyrate dehydrogenase (HBD) as an indirect measure of LDH_1 and LDH_2.

CPK—creatine phosphokinase, found in the heart, skeletal muscle, and brain, but not in red blood cells or the liver. CPK levels rise after strenuous exercise, polymyositis, muscular dystrophy, muscle injury, and MI. After skeletal muscle abnormalities and cerebral disease are ruled out, *elevated CPK is considered specific for myocardial damage.* Intramuscular injections *alone* can elevate the CPK enzyme level. Some laboratories solve this problem by separating CPK into the isoenzymes CPK_1, or BB (brain tissues); CPK_2, or MB (heart muscle); and CPK_3, or MM (skeletal muscle).

When CPK is separated, *all* of the total CPK value should be CPK_3, or MM. If CPK_2, or MB, is present, it is indicative of myocardial damage, which always elevates the CPK value. A positive MB value with EKG changes is positive identification of an MI.

Controllable Factors in Coronary Artery Disease

Hypertension greatly predisposes to coronary artery disease. The risk of coronary artery disease increases sharply as diastolic blood pressure exceeds 90 mm Hg and the systolic exceeds 140 mm Hg. In uncontrolled hypertension, the heart must work harder to force blood from the left ventricle into the constricted peripheral circuit. Consequently, the myocardium hypertrophies, needing much more oxygen to energize the greater muscle mass of the left ventricle. Controlling blood pressure requires control of obesity, restricted salt intake, and the careful use of diuretics and antihypertensives. Uncontrolled hypertension commonly results from late diagnosis or poor compliance with recommended treatment.

Diabetes is another source of circulatory damage. Controlling it through diet and insulin helps to reduce connective tissue degeneration, which may accelerate atherogenesis; and to regulate body insulin, which may affect lipid metabolism and arterial response.

Diet may affect one risk factor, hyperlipidemia. High levels of cholesterol, triglyceride, and saturated fatty acids have been linked with increased coronary artery disease. We can recommend moderation in daily fat intake (using more polyunsaturated than saturated fats) and control of obesity. Probably the best course of action is to encourage regular, vigorous physical activity to use up those ingested fats.

Smoking overstimulates the heart, constricts peripheral blood vessels, and releases carbon monoxide, which interferes with myocardial oxygenation.

Sedentary life-style is a risk factor for coronary heart disease. Regular exercise offers many proven benefits: reduction in heart rate, systolic blood pressure, blood lipids, and body weight; and increases in exercise tolerance, cardiac efficiency, fibrinolytic activity, and overall well-being. However, regular exercise doesn't always mean all will be well.

Stress may aggravate coronary artery disease.

No one can totally avoid stress, but patients can learn to reduce stress by avoiding noise and crowds; by changing stressful jobs; by learning to accept what cannot be changed; by exercising to release tension (yoga, walking, or just deep-breathing exercises); by getting adequate rest and sleep; and by developing an enjoyable hobby.

Coronary Artery Disease (CAD)

Description
• Decreased coronary blood flow, reducing the amount of oxygen and essential nutrients delivered to myocardial tissue
• More common in men than in women and in whites, the middle-aged, and the elderly

Possible causes
• Atherosclerosis most common cause; less commonly results from dissecting aneurysm, infectious vasculitis, syphilis, and congenital defects

Signs and symptoms
• Burning, squeezing, or crushing pain in substernal or precordial chest that may radiate to left arm, neck, jaws, or shoulder blade
• Anginal episodes following physical exertion, emotional excitement, or temperature changes
• Patient describes pain by clenching fist over chest or rubbing left arm
• Nausea
• Vomiting
• Faintness
• Diaphoresis
• Cool extremities

Nursing intervention
• During anginal episodes, monitor blood pressure and heart rate. Take an EKG before administering nitroglycerin or other nitrates. Note duration of pain, amount of medication required to relieve it, and accompanying symptoms.

• Have nitroglycerin on hand for immediate use. Instruct the patient to notify you immediately whenever he feels chest pain and takes nitroglycerin.
• Prepare the patient for cardiac catheterization by explaining the procedure to him and making sure he knows why it is necessary, understands the risk involved, and realizes that its results may indicate a need for surgery.
• After the catheterization, review the expected course of treatment with the patient and his family. Monitor the catheter site (usually the antecubital fossa or groin) for bleeding. Also check pulses distal to the catheter insertion site. To counter the diuretic effect of the dye used for the test, make sure the patient drinks plenty of fluids. To prevent dysrhythmias from muscle irritability, monitor potassium levels closely.
• If the patient is scheduled for surgery, explain the procedure to the patient and his family and answer their questions.
• Emphasize to your patient the importance of taking his medication exactly as prescribed, exercising regularly, and observing any dietary restrictions.
• Stress the need to stop smoking. Refer the patient to a self-help group if necessary.

Heart Failure: Nursing Intervention

CARDIOVASCULAR DISORDERS

• Schedule the patient for an EKG to detect heart strain and ischemia.
• Arrange for the patient to have a chest X-ray to detect heart enlargement, increased pulmonary marking, interstitial edema, and pleural effusion and cardiomegaly.
• Measure the patient for antiembolism stockings, as ordered. Teach him how to apply the stockings.
• Encourage bed rest, as ordered.
• Administer vasodilators, such as prazosin hydrochloride (Minipress*), as ordered.
• Instruct the patient to weigh himself daily at the same time in similar clothing. Tell him to notify you if he gains 1 lb (0.4 kg) or more a day for 3 consecutive days.
• Advise the patient to avoid foods high in sodium content, such as canned or commercially prepared foods, and to avoid dairy products to curb fluid overload. Tell him not to add salt to his food.
• Explain to the patient that he must replace the potassium lost through diuretics by taking a potassium supplement and by eating high-potassium foods such as bananas, apricots, and orange juice.
• Stress the need for frequent checkups.

• Emphasize the importance of taking digitalis exactly as prescribed. Instruct the patient to watch for signs of digitalis toxicity.
• Teach the patient how to take his own pulse. Have him notify you or the doctor if his pulse rate is unusually irregular or is less than 160 beats/minute; if he experiences dizziness, blurred vision, shortness of breath, a persistent, dry cough, palpitations, increased fatigue, paroxysmal nocturnal dyspnea, swollen ankles, decreased urinary output; or if he gains 3 to 5 lb (1.36 to 2.20 kg) in a week.
• Tell the patient to avoid fatigue by pacing activities, simplifying his workload, and obtaining help from others.
• Teach the patient methods of promoting proper respiratory function, such as getting adequate rest, elevating the head of the bed, limiting exposure to extreme temperature conditions, providing adequate indoor humidity, avoiding persons with respiratory tract infections, and being immunized against influenza.
• Instruct the patient or his family to report signs of unusual fatigue, respiratory status changes, weight gain, or confusion to you or the doctor.

*Also available in Canada

Conditions Affecting Pump Action

LEFT VENTRICULAR FAILURE

Chief complaint
- *Chest pain:* usually absent
- *Dyspnea:* present on exertion, accompanied by cough, orthopnea, paroxysmal nocturnal dyspnea; in advanced disease, present at rest
- *Fatigue:* present on exertion, accompanied by weakness
- *Irregular heartbeat:* may be present; patient may complain of rapid heart rate and skipped beats

History
- Patient uses pillow to prop self up for sleep; wakes up gasping for breath; must sit or stand for relief
- History of present illness includes wheezing on inspiration and expiration (cardiac asthma), right upper abdominal pain or discomfort on exertion, daytime oliguria, nighttime polyuria, constipation (uncommon), anorexia, progressive weight gain, generalized edema, progressive weakness, fatigue, decreased mentation
- Past medical history includes severe chronic congestive heart failure

Physical examination
- Inspection reveals profuse sweating, pallor, cyanosis, frothy white or pink sputum, heaving apical impulse, hand veins that remain distended when patient puts hands above level of right atrium
- Palpation reveals enlarged, diffuse, and sustained left ventricular impulse at precordium

Diagnostic Studies
- Pulmonary artery and pulmonary capillary wedge pressures elevated
- Central venous pressure elevated if condition has advanced to right ventricular failure, or hypervolemia from increased sodium and water retention
- EKG reflects heart strain or left ventricular enlargement, ischemia, and dysrhythmias
- X-ray shows left atrial enlargement and pulmonary venous congestion

CARDIOVASCULAR DISORDERS

Continued

Conditions Affecting Pump Action
Continued

CARDIOVASCULAR
DISORDERS

ACUTE RIGHT VENTRICU-LAR FAILURE

Chief complaint
• *Chest pain:* usually absent
• *Dyspnea:* respiratory distress secondary to pulmonary disease or advanced left ventricular failure
• *Fatigue:* in severe cases, weakness and mental aberration
• *Irregular heartbeat:* atrial dysrhythmias common
• *Peripheral changes:* dependent edema: begins in ankles but progresses to legs and genitalia; initially subsides at night, later does not; ascites; weight gain
History
• History of present illness includes anorexia, right upper abdominal pain or discomfort during exertion, nausea, and vomiting
• Past medical history includes left ventricular failure, mitral stenosis, pulmonic valve stenosis, tricuspid regurgitation, pulmonary hypertension, chronic obstructive pulmonary disease

Physical examination
• Inspection reveals lower sternal or left parasternal heave independent of apical impulse
• Palpation and percussion reveal enlarged, tender, pulsating liver, with tricuspid regurgitation; abdomen fluid wave and shifting dullness; hepatojugular reflex, indicating jugular vein distention; tachycardia
• Auscultation reveals right ventricular S_3 sound; murmur of tricuspid regurgitation
Diagnostic studies
• Central venous pressure readings are elevated

CARDIOMYOPATHIES

Chief complaint
• *Dyspnea:* paroxysmal nocturnal, accompanied by orthopnea
• *Fatigue:* present
• *Irregular heartbeat:* palpitations; Stokes-Adams attacks with conduction defects
• *Peripheral changes:* dry skin, extremity pain, edema, ascites with right-sided failure

Continued

Conditions Affecting Pump Action
Continued

CARDIOMYOPATHIES
Continued

History
• Past medical history includes viral illness, alcoholism, chronic debilitating illnesses

Physical examination
• Fever
• Signs of right and/or left heart failure
• Palpation reveals displaced cardiac impulse to left tachycardia
• Auscultation reveals systolic murmur, S_3 sound, and postural hypotension

Diagnostic studies
• EKG reveals nonspecific ST-T changes, decreased height of R wave; may show dysrhythmias and conduction defects (especially atrial fibrillation)
• Echocardiography and chest X-ray may help determine heart size

IDIOPATHIC HYPERTRO-
PHIC SUBAORTIC STENO-
SIS (IHSS)

Chief complaint
• *Chest pain:* present; similar to angina pectoris, but unrelieved by nitroglycerin
• *Dyspnea:* present on exertion
• *Fatigue:* present; along with dizziness and syncope
• *Irregular heartbeat:* may be present; patient may complain of palpitations or skipped beats
• *Peripheral changes:* peripheral edema (uncommon)

History
• Symptoms may be induced by high temperatures, pregnancy, exercise, standing suddenly, Valsalva's maneuver

Physical examination
• Palpation reveals peripheral pulse with characteristic double impulse
• Auscultation reveals systolic ejection murmur
• In advanced stage, signs of mitral insufficiency (such as systolic murmur), congestive heart failure, and sudden death possible

Continued

Conditions Affecting Pump Action
Continued

IDIOPATHIC HYPERTRO-
PHIC SUBAORTIC STENO-
SIS (IHSS)
Continued

Diagnostic studies
● EKG reveals left ventricular hypertrophy, ST segment, and T wave abnormalities
● Echocardiography shows increased interventricular system thickness and abnormal mitral valve motion

PERICARDITIS

Chief complaint
● *Chest pain:* sudden onset; precordial or substernal, pleuritic, radiating to left neck, shoulder, back, or epigastrium; worsened by lying down or swallowing
History
● Past medical history includes viral respiratory infection, recent pericardiotomy or myocardial infarction, disseminated lupus erythematosus, serum sickness, acute rheumatic fever, trauma, uremia, lymphoma

● Most common in men between ages 20 and 50
Physical examination
● Fever: 100° to 103° F. (37.8° to 39.4° C.)
● Palpation reveals tachycardia
● Auscultation reveals pericardial friction rub
Diagnostic studies
● EKG shows ST-T segment elevation in all leads; returns to baseline in a few days, with T wave inversion
● Possibly atrial fibrillation

PERICARDITIS WITH EFFUSION

Chief complaint
● *Chest pain:* may be present as dull, diffuse precordial or substernal distress
● *Dyspnea:* present; associated with cough that causes patient to lean forward for relief
● *Peripheral changes:* none
History
● Past medical history includes uremia, malignancy, connective tissue disorder, viral pericarditis

Continued

Conditions Affecting Pump Action
Continued

PERICARDITIS WITH EFFUSION
Continued

Physical examination
• Inspection reveals distended neck veins
• Palpation and percussion reveal tachycardia, enlarged area of cardiac dullness, apical beat that's within dullness border or not palpable
• Auscultation reveals abnormal blood pressure and possibly pericardial friction rub, and acute cardiac tamponade; may progress to shock

Diagnostic studies
• EKG shows T waves flat, low diphasic or inverted leads, QRS voltage uniformly low

SUBACUTE AND ACUTE INFECTIVE ENDOCARDITIS

Chief complaint
• *Chest pain:* present; also in abdomen, and in flanks (uncommon)
• *Dyspnea:* present in approximately 50% of cases; depends on severity of disease or valve involved

• *Fatigue:* present, usually as malaise
• *Irregular heartbeat:* absent
• *Peripheral changes:* weight loss, redness or swelling, heart failure symptoms

History
• Present or recent history includes acute infection, surgery or instrumentation, dental work, drug abuse, abortion, transurethral prostatectomy
• Past medical history includes rheumatic, congenital, or artherosclerotic heart disease

Physical examination
• Daily fever
• Inspection may show petechiae on conjunctivae and palate buccal mucosa, with long-standing endocarditis; clubbed fingers and toes; splinter hemorrhages under nails; tender red nodules on finger and toe pads; pallor or yellow-brown skin; oval, pale, retinal lesion around optic disk
• Palpation reveals splenomegaly
• Auscultation reveals sudden change in present heart murmur or development of new

Continued

Conditions Affecting Pump Action
Continued

CARDIOVASCULAR
DISORDERS

SUBACUTE AND ACUTE INFECTIVE ENDOCARDITIS
Continued

murmur and possibly signs of early heart failure or emboli
Diagnostic studies
• Blood cultures determine causative organism
• Echocardiograph—particularly the two-dimensional (2-D) method—looks for vegetation

RHEUMATIC FEVER (acute)

Chief complaint
• *Chest pain:* absent
• *Dyspnea:* may be present
• *Fatigue:* malaise
• *Irregular heartbeat:* absent
• *Peripheral changes:* weight loss
History
• Recent history includes streptococcal infection of upper respiratory tract (in previous 4 weeks), anorexia
• Past medical history includes migratory, gradually beginning arthritis; recurrent epistaxis; "growing pains" in joints (arthralgia)

• Increased clumsiness
Physical examination
• Usually low-grade fever, with sinus tachycardia disproportional to fever level
• Inspection reveals erythema marginatum (ring- or crescent-shaped macular rash), subcutaneous nodules (uncommon except in children), swollen joints (arthritis), Sydenham's chorea
• Palpation reveals enlarged heart
• Auscultation reveals mitral or aortic diastolic murmurs, varying heart sound quality, and possibly gallop rhythm, dysrhythmias and ectopic beats
Diagnostic studies
• Erythrocyte sedimentation rate and WBC count elevated.
• Throat cultures positive for beta-hemolytic streptococci
• Antistreptolysin titer elevated
• Chest X-ray may show cardiac enlargement
• EKG shows PR greater than 0.2 seconds; may further define dysrhythmias

Conditions Affecting Valvular Function

TRICUSPID STENOSIS

Chief complaint
• *Chest pain:* usually absent
• *Dyspnea:* present in varying degrees
• *Fatigue:* present; often severe
• *Irregular heartbeat:* usually absent
• *Peripheral changes:* dependent peripheral edema
History
• Most common in women
• Past medical history includes mitral valve disease
Physical examination
• Inspection may reveal olive skin
• Palpation may reveal presystolic liver pulsation if in sinus rhythm; middiastolic thrill between lower left sternal border and apical impulse
• Auscultation reveals diastolic rumbling murmur heard along lower left sternal border; normal blood pressure
Diagnostic studies
• EKG shows wide, tall, peaked P waves; normal axis
• Echocardiography may permit stenosis recognition

• X-ray shows enlarged right atrium
• Cardiac catheterization may reveal site of stenosis

TRICUSPID REGURGITATION (incompetence)

Chief complaint
• *Chest pain:* absent
• *Dyspnea:* present
• *Fatigue:* present
• *Irregular heartbeat:* atrial fibrillation; usually not noticed by patient
• *Peripheral changes:* none
History
• Past medical history includes right ventricular failure, rheumatic fever, trauma, endocarditis, pulmonary hypertension
Physical examination
• Palpation reveals right ventricular pulsation
• Auscultation reveals blowing, coarse, or harsh systolic murmur heard along lower left sternal border; increases on inspiration
Diagnostic studies
• EKG usually shows atrial fibrillation   *Continued*

CARDIOVASCULAR DISORDERS

Conditions Affecting Valvular Function
Continued

AORTIC STENOSIS

Chief complaint
- *Chest pain:* present in severe stenosis
- *Dyspnea:* present, with coughing, on exertion; paroxysmal nocturnal
- *Fatigue:* usually present; syncope
- *Irregular heartbeat:* present, as palpitations occasionally

History
- Most common in males
- Usually asymptomatic unless severe

Physical examination
- Inspection reveals apical impulse localized and heaving, usually not laterally displaced
- Palpation reveals sustained, localized, forceful apical impulse; systolic thrill over aortic area and neck vessels; small, slowly rising plateau pulse, best appreciated in carotid pulse
- Auscultation reveals harsh, rough, systolic ejection murmur in aortic area, radiating to the neck and apex; possibly systolic ejection click at aortic area just before murmur; paradoxical splitting of second sound with significant stenosis; normal or high diastolic blood pressure

Diagnostic studies
- EKG shows criteria for left ventricular hypertrophy; possibly complete heart block
- X-rays and fluoroscopy may show calcified aortic valve, poststenotic dilatation of ascending aorta (hyperactivity evident with fluoroscopy), left ventricular hypertrophy
- Echocardiography may identify level of obstruction and a bicuspid aortic valve
- Cardiac catheterization indicates the severity and location of the obstruction as well as left ventricular function

AORTIC REGURGITATION
(incompetence)

Chief complaint
- *Chest pain:* angina pectoris
- *Dyspnea:* on exertion early in disease; paroxysmal nocturnal dyspnea; orthopnea and cough signal beginning of decompensation

Continued

Conditions Affecting Valvular Function
Continued

AORTIC REGURGITATION
(incompetence)
Continued

• *Fatigue:* present; weakness if left ventricular failure present
• *Irregular heartbeat:* palpitations
History
• Past medical history includes Reiter's syndrome, rheumatoid arthritis, psoriasis, rheumatic fever, syphilis, infective endocarditis
Physical examination
• Inspection reveals generalized skin pallor; strong carotid pulsations; forceful apical impulse to left of left midclavicular line and downward
• Palpation reveals sustained, forceful apical impulse; rapidly rising and collapsing pulses
• Auscultation reveals normal heart sounds; soft, blowing, diastolic murmur; in advanced aortic insufficiency, Austin Flint murmur may be heard at apex; with diastolic pressure less than 60 mm Hg

Diagnostic studies
• EKG shows evidence of left ventricular hypertrophy
• X-ray shows enlarged left ventricle
• Echocardiography shows aortic valve incompetence
• Cardiac catheterization performed to exclude complicating lesions and to assess left ventricular function

MITRAL STENOSIS

Chief complaint
• *Chest pain:* usually absent
• *Dyspnea:* present; may also occur during rest; orthopnea; paroxysmal nocturnal dyspnea; hemoptysis
• *Fatigue:* present; increased with decreased exercise tolerance
• *Irregular heartbeat:* usually absent
• *Peripheral changes:* extremity pain
History
• Most common in women under age 45
• Recent bronchitis or upper respiratory tract infection may worsen symptoms

Continued

CARDIOVASCULAR
DISORDERS

Conditions Affecting Valvular Function
Continued

MITRAL STENOSIS
Continued

- Past medical history includes rheumatic fever, congenital valve disorder, tumor (myxoma)

Physical examination
- Inspection reveals malar flush; in young patients, precordial bulge and diffuse pulsation
- Palpation reveals tapping sensation over area of expected apical impulse, mid-diastolic and/or presystolic thrill at apex, small pulse, overactive right ventricle with elevated pulmonary pressure
- Auscultation reveals localized, delayed, rumbling, low-pitched, diastolic murmur at or near apex (duration of murmur varies depending on severity of stenosis); possibly loud S_2 with elevated pulmonary pressure; normal blood pressure

Diagnostic studies
- EKG shows notched and broad P waves in standard leads; inverted P in V_1 lead; atrial fibrillation common
- X-ray and fluoroscopy show left atrial enlargement
- Echocardiography helps assess severity of stenosis
- Cardiac catheterization and angiocardiography help determine amount of regurgitation that may also be present

MITRAL REGURGITATION
(incompetence)

Chief complaint
- *Chest pain:* absent
- *Dyspnea:* present, progressive with exertion; orthopnea, paroxysmal dyspnea
- *Fatigue:* present, progressive with exertion
- *Irregular heartbeat:* present as palpitations
- *Peripheral changes:* none

History
- Past medical history includes rheumatic fever, endocarditis, congenital mitral valve defect, papillary muscle dysfunction or rupture, chordae tendinae dysfunction or rupture, heart failure associated with left ventricular dilation, blunt injury to the chest

Physical examination
- Inspection reveals forceful apical impulse to left of left midclavicular line

Continued

Conditions Affecting Valvular Function
Continued

MITRAL REGURGITATION
(incompetence)
Continued

- Palpation reveals brisk apical impulse; systolic thrill over apical impulse; normal or slightly collapsing pulse
- Auscultation reveals blowing, high-pitched, harsh, or musical pansystolic apical murmur maximal at apex and transmitted to axilla; abnormally wide splitting of S_2; normal blood pressure

Diagnostic studies
- EKG shows P waves broad or notched in standard leads; with pulmonary hypertension, tall peaked P waves, right axis deviation, or right ventricular hypertrophy; possibly atrial fibrillation
- X-ray shows enlargement of left ventricle and moderate aneurysmal dilatation of left atrium
- Echocardiography shows dilated left ventricle and left atrium
- Cardiac catheterization and ventriculography help determine amount of regurgitation and identify prolapsing cusps

PULMONIC STENOSIS

Chief complaint
- *Chest pain:* usually none
- *Dyspnea:* present on exertion
- *Fatigue:* present
- *Peripheral changes:* peripheral edema possible

History
- Congenital stenosis or rheumatic heart disease, associated with other congenital heart defects

Physical examination
- Inspection reveals jugular vein distention
- Palpation reveals hepatomegaly
- Auscultation reveals systolic murmur at left sternal border and split S_2 sound

Diagnostic studies
- EKG shows right ventricular hypertrophy, right axis deviation, right atrial hypertrophy

PULMONIC REGURGITATION
(incompetence)

Chief complaint
- *Chest pain:* absent

Continued

Conditions Affecting Valvular Function
Continued

PULMONIC REGURGITA-
TION (incompetence)
Continued

- *Dyspnea:* present
- *Fatigue:* present; patient
tires easily; weakness
- *Irregular heartbeat:* absent
- *Peripheral changes:* periph-
eral edema
History
- Pulmonary hypertension

- Congenital defect
Physical examination
- Inspection reveals jugular
vein distention
- Palpation reveals hepato-
megaly
- Auscultation reveals dia-
stolic murmur in pulmonic
area
Diagnostic studies
- EKG shows right ventricular
or right atrial enlargement

Managing Valvular Function Disorders

Treatment of valvular function disorders depends on the nature and
severity of associated symptoms.
For example, heart failure requires digoxin, diuretics, a so-
dium-restricted diet, and in acute
cases, oxygen. Atrial fibrillation
requires digoxin or electrical con-
version, and if pulmonary edema
occurs, oxygen and I.V. administration of diuretics.

If the patient has severe symptoms that can't be managed med-
ically, open heart surgery using
cardiopulmonary bypass for valve
replacement is indicated. Other
appropriate measures include an-
ticoagulant therapy to prevent
thrombus formation around dis-

eased or replaced valves, and
prophylactic antibiotics before and
after surgery or dental care.
- Watch closely for signs of heart
failure or pulmonary edema, and
side effects of drug therapy.
- Teach the patient about diet restrictions, medications, symptoms
that should be reported, and the
importance of consistent follow-up
care.
- If the patient undergoes surgery, watch for hypotension, dysrhythmias, and thrombus formation. Monitor vital signs, arterial
blood gases, intake and output,
daily weight, blood chemistries,
chest X-rays, and pulmonary artery catheter readings.

Guide to Cardiopulmonary Emergencies

Do you know what emergency care to give in the following cardio-pulmonary emergencies? The chart below will give you specific instructions. Study them carefully. In addition, remember these guidelines that apply to every cardiopulmonary emergency:

Call the doctor immediately. Make sure the patient has an open airway. Monitor him closely for signs of shock, and begin I.V. therapy, as needed, with the appropriate solution. Draw blood for type and cross-matching in case your patient needs a blood transfusion. Get a complete medical history from the patient or his family, including information about the accident or injury (when applicable).

CARDIAC CONTUSION

Problem/Signs and symptoms
• History of injury to anterior chest
• Ecchymosis on chest wall
• Retrosternal angina, unrelieved by nitroglycerin, but sometimes relieved by O_2 therapy
• Tachycardia
• EKG reading indicating *apparent* myocardial infarction or conduction disturbances
• Pericardial friction rub
• *Important:* in some cases, patient with a cardiac contusion may be asymptomatic

Special emergency nursing considerations
• Follow the general guidelines listed above
• Stay alert for signs of a ruptured aorta or ventricle; also watch for signs of cardiac tamponade
• Prepare patient for admission to the hospital; the doctor will want him to have continuous EKG monitoring

PENETRATING WOUND IN HEART

Problem/Signs and symptoms
• In most cases, patient has a visible chest wound caused by object like knife or bullet; however, heart penetration can occur from a bullet entering the abdomen or back
• Chest pain, bleeding
• Drowsiness, loss of consciousness, possible agitation, combativeness, or confusion (Note: patient may appear intoxicated)
• Tachycardia, muffled heart

Continued

Guide to Cardiopulmonary Emergencies
Continued

PENETRATING WOUND IN HEART
Continued

sounds, hypotension, dyspnea, increased central venous pressure (CVP)
• Distended neck veins, although these may not be present immediately; for example, if the patient's in hypovolemic shock from blood loss, he may not have neck vein distention until he receives adequate I.V. fluid replacement
• Pneumothorax or hemothorax
Special emergency nursing considerations
• Follow the general guidelines listed on page 95.
• If a penetrating object is still in place when the patient arrives in the emergency department, don't remove it; let it be a seal for the damaged blood vessels and heart
• Place the patient on cardiac monitor
• If the penetrating object's already been removed, control bleeding by applying di-

ect pressure to the wound with a sterile cloth
• Administer oxygen; be prepared to intubate patient.
• If the doctor decides to insert a chest tube, be ready to assist
• Prepare the patient for a thoracotomy

RUPTURED AORTA

Problem/Signs and symptoms
• History of abrupt deceleration or compression injury
• Chest or back pain
• Dyspnea; weak, thready pulse; weakness in extremities; drowsiness, loss of consciousness
• Increased blood pressure and pulse amplitude in upper extremities, and decreased blood pressure and pulse amplitude in lower extremities
Special emergency nursing considerations
• Follow the general guidelines listed on page 95.
• Prepare patient for immediate surgery

Continued

Guide to Cardiopulmonary Emergencies
Continued

RUPTURED AORTA
Continued

- Administer oxygen and place patient on cardiac monitor
- Have emergency equipment nearby
- Get ready to administer nitroprusside (Nipride), according to doctor's order.
- When you monitor patient's vital signs, pay particular attention to the pulses in his legs

CARDIAC TAMPONADE

Problem/Signs and symptoms
(a condition in which fluid or blood becomes trapped between the heart muscle and the pericardial sac)
- History of blunt trauma to anterior chest, penetrating chest wound, or recent cardiac surgery. *Important:* Tamponade may also be a complication of a medical problem; for example, pericardial neoplasm or uremia. Tamponade may also follow cardiac catheterization, pacemaker insertion, or pericardiocentesis.
- Dyspnea, possible cyanosis, agitation, and neck vein distention
- Weak, thready pulse or paradoxical pulse in which blood pressure drops on inspiration
- Absent third heart sound
- Hypotension with narrowed pulse pressure
- Increased central venous pressure (CVP)
- Decreased urinary output

Special emergency nursing considerations
- Follow the general guidelines listed on page 95.
- Prepare to assist the doctor with a pericardiocentesis; assemble the needed equipment.
- Place patient on cardiac monitor
- Administer oxygen
- Following pericardiocentesis, prepare patient for a thoracotomy; as you do, observe him closely for recurring signs of tamponade, which may result in cardiac arrest
- Watch for signs of pulmonary emboli: extreme agitation, dyspnea, pallor, combativeness, chest pain; notify doctor immediately

CARDIOVASCULAR DISORDERS

What Happens in Cardiac Tamponade

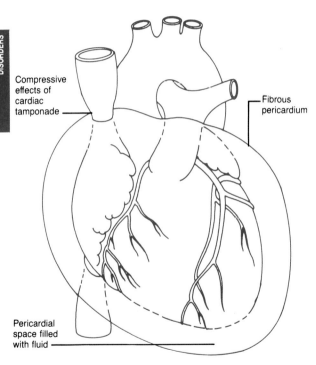

Compressive effects of cardiac tamponade

Fibrous pericardium

Pericardial space filled with fluid

Monitoring Your Patient During Emergency Pericardiocentesis

If the doctor suspects your patient has cardiac tamponade, he may perform emergency pericardiocentesis. (This procedure is also used to diagnose pericardial effusion.) Pericardiocentesis involves inserting a 16G to 18G intracardiac needle into the pericardial sac to aspirate fluid and to relieve intrapericardial pressure.

Pericardiocentesis may cause life-threatening complications, such as ventricular dysrhythmias, bleeding from the myocardium, and coronary artery laceration. A precordial lead, attached to the needle's hub, lets the EKG monitor reflect needle position. If the needle contacts the patient's myocardium inadvertently, causing bleeding and ventricular irritability, you'll see abnormal wave forms—large and erratic QRS complexes. Elevated ST segments indicate that the needle's contacted the ventricle; prolonged PR intervals indicate that it's touched the atrium.

Instruct the patient why the test is being performed. Tell him that a local anesthetic will be injected before the aspiration needle is put in place. Also, make sure he realizes that he'll experience pressure when the needle's inserted.

If time allows, review the patient's history of antibiotic usage and record this information on the request form.

During the test, monitor your patient's EKG, blood pressure, and central venous pressure (CVP) constantly. Be alert for grossly bloody aspirate. This ominous sign may indicate inadvertent puncture of a cardiac chamber. Make sure, too, that emergency resuscitation equipment's on hand.

Following the procedure, monitor your patient's vital signs every 5 to 10 minutes. His blood pressure should rise as the tamponade's relieved.

Be alert for signs and symptoms of recurring tamponade (which may require repeated pericardiocentesis):
• decreased blood pressure
• narrowing pulse pressure
• increased CVP
• distended neck veins
• tachycardia
• tachypnea
• muffled heart sounds
• friction rub
• anxiety
• chest pain.

Peripheral Circulation Disorders

VARICOSE VEINS

Chief complaints
- *Chest pain:* absent
- *Peripheral changes:* aching discomfort or pain in legs; pigmentation and ulceration of distal leg; possibly edema

History
- History of present illness includes leg cramps at night that may be relieved by leg elevation, itching in vein regions, leg fatigue caused by periods of standing
- Past medical history includes thrombophlebitis and family history of varicosities

Physical examination/Diagnostic studies
- Inspection reveals dilated tortuous vessels in legs, visible when patient stands; brown pigmentation and thinning of skin above ankles; ulceration of distal leg; positive Trendelenburg's test
- No diagnostic studies usually performed

THROMBOPHLEBITIS

Chief complaints
- *Chest pain:* present with pulmonary embolism
- *Peripheral changes:* pain and swelling of affected extremity; if leg veins affected, pain may increase with walking

History
- Childbirth 4 to 14 days before onset
- History of present illness includes fracture, trauma, deep vein surgery, cardiac disease, cerebrovascular accident, prolonged bed rest
- Past medical history includes malignancy, shock, dehydration anemia, obesity, chronic infection, use of oral contraceptives
- In superficial vein thrombophlebitis, recent history includes superficial vein I.V. therapy with irritating solutions

Physical examination/Diagnostic studies
- Slight fever
- In deep vein involvement, severe venous obstruction is revealed by cyanotic skin in affected area; reflex arterial spasm, by pale and cool skin
- Palpation reveals warm affected leg, spasm and pain in calf muscles with dorsiflexion of foot (positive Homans' sign)
- In superficial vein involvement, inspection reveals induration, redness, tenderness along course of vein; possibly no clinical manifestations
- Ultrasound blood flow detector, thermography, and phlebography used to confirm diagnosis

Continued

Peripheral Circulation Disorders
Continued

DISSECTING THORACIC AOR-
TIC ANEURYSMS

Chief complaints
• *Chest pain:* present; sudden
and severe, radiating to back, abdomen, and hips
• *Peripheral changes:* paralysis of
legs possible
History
• Recent history may include convulsions
• Past medical history includes
hypertension, arteriosclerosis,
congenital heart disease, Mar-
fan's syndrome, pregnancy,
trauma
Physical examination/Diagnos-
tic studies
• Fever
• Palpation reveals unequal or diminished peripheral pulses
• Auscultation reveals aortic diastolic murmur and murmurs over
arteries
• Aortography shows size and extent of aneurysm

ABDOMINAL AORTIC ANEU-
RYSM

Chief complaints
• *Chest pain:* absent
• *Peripheral changes:* absent
History
• Usually in men over age 50

Physical examination/Diagnos-
tic studies
• Inspection reveals subcutaneous ecchymosis in flank or
groin
• Palpation reveals pulsating mid-
abdominal and upper abdominal
mass
• Aortography shows size of
aneurysm
• EKG, urinalysis, blood urea ni-
trogen evaluate renal and cardiac
function

RAYNAUD'S DISEASE AND
RAYNAUD'S PHENOMENON

Chief complaints
• *Chest pain:* absent
• *Peripheral changes:* with Raynaud's disease: attacks of cyanosis, followed by pallor in fingers
(rarely, in thumbs or toes); redness, swelling, throbbing, and
paresthesia during recovery, occurring when areas are warmed;
numbness, stiffness, diminished
sensation; with Raynaud's phenomenon: usually unilateral cyanosis, which may involve only one
or two fingers
History
• Most common in females between puberty and age 40
• Precipitating factors include
emotional upsets or a cold
• Past history includes immuno-
logic abnormalities   *Continued*

Peripheral Circulation Disorders
Continued

RAYNAUD'S DISEASE AND
RAYNAUD'S PHENOMENON
Continued

• Family history of vasospastic diseases
• Raynaud's phenomenon may accompany cervical rib, carpal tunnel syndrome, scleroderma,

systemic lupus erythematosus, frostbite, ergot poisoning
Physical examination/Diagnostic studies
• Inspection reveals atrophy of terminal fat pads of fingers
• No diagnostic studies usually performed

Peripheral Arterial Disease: What Patients Need to Know

Peripheral arterial disease causes the walls of large and medium-sized peripheral arteries to thicken, harden, and lose their elasticity. As the lumen narrows, the blood flow decreases and blood clots may form. When collateral circulation cannot compensate for the block, ischemia results. The patient with arteriosclerosis, age 50 or older, will feel a viselike pain during exercise, distal to the blockage. In advanced cases, pain may occur even during rest.

Have your patients with arteriosclerosis follow this checklist of do's and don'ts:
DO:
• Stop smoking.
• Wash feet daily and wear clean, well-fitting socks.
• Trim nails straight across but

not too closely.
• Clean small cuts carefully with mild soap and water, and protect from further injury.
• Call the doctor to report any persistent leg problem.
DON'T:
• Don't go barefoot.
• Don't let your legs become extremely cold.
• Don't wear clothes that constrict your legs or feet.
• Don't let your legs get sunburned.
• Don't cut or file corns or calluses. Don't use chemical corn and callus remedies.
• Don't put a hot water bottle, heat lamp, or heating pad directly on the affected area. Instead, put the heat on the lower back or abdomen. This will warm the legs in about 15 minutes.

Miscellaneous Code Drugs

ATROPINE SULFATE

Dose and route
For AV block, junctional or escape rhythms, severe nodal or sinus bradycardia: 0.5 to 1.0 mg I.V. bolus.
Interactions
None significant.
Possible side effects
Dry mouth, mental confusion, palpitations, urinary retention, tachycardia
Special considerations
• Monitor heart rate and rhythm to determine the drug's effects. Doses lower than 0.5 mg can cause paradoxical bradycardia. Store drug in amber or light-resistant container. Dose may be repeated q 5 minutes up to 2 mg.

CALCIUM CHLORIDE

Dose and route
For asystole: 0.5 to 1 g I.V. bolus.
Interactions
Cardiac glycosides: increased digitalis toxicity; administer calcium very cautiously, if at all, to digitalized patients.

Possible side effects
Bradycardia, hypercalcemia, syncope, tingling sensations
Special considerations
• Monitor EKG when giving calcium I.V. Such injections should not exceed 0.7 to 1.5 mEq/minute. Stop if patient complains of discomfort.
• Report abnormalities.
• Hypercalcemia may result after large doses in chronic renal failure.
• If possible, administer I.V. into a large vein.
• I.V. route generally recommended in children, but not by scalp vein.
• Solutions should be warmed to body temperature before administration.
• Calcium chloride should be given I.V. only.
• Severe necrosis and sloughing of tissues follow extravasation. Calcium gluconate is less irritating to veins and tissues than calcium chloride.
• Following injection, patient should be recumbent for 15 minutes.
• Crash carts usually contain

Continued

TREATMENT

Miscellaneous Code Drugs
Continued

CALCIUM CHLORIDE
Continued

both gluconate and chloride. Make sure doctor specifies form he wants administered.

MAGNESIUM SULFATE

Dose and route
Adults: 1 g (8 mEq) I.V. slow push over 1 minute (2 ml of 50% solution). May repeat after 5 minutes if no response.
Contraindications
• Use cautiously in patients with impaired renal function, myocardial damage, and heart block, and in women in labor.
Possible side effects
Sweating, depressed reflexes, hypotension, flushing, circulatory collapse, heart block, respiratory paralysis
Special considerations
• Monitor vital signs every 15 minutes when administering
• Check magnesium blood levels after repeated doses. Disappearance of knee-jerk and patellar reflexes is a sign of pending magnesium toxicity.

SODIUM BICARBONATE

Indications
• Cardiac arrest
• Metabolic acidosis
Dosage
Adults
Cardiac arrest
I.V. bolus: 1 to 3 mEq/kg, initially; followed by 0.5 mEq/kg q 10 minutes depending on blood gases. Further dose based on arterial blood gas (ABG) measurement.
Metabolic acidosis
I.V. infusion: 2 to 5 mEq over a 4- to 8-hour period.
Children
Cardiac arrest
I.V. bolus: 1 mEq/kg. Further dose based on ABG measurement. Not to exceed 8 mEq/kg/day.
Contraindications
• No contraindications for life-threatening emergencies.
• Contraindicated in patients with hypertension, renal disease, tendency toward edema, in those losing chlorides by vomiting or from continuous GI suction, in those receiving diuretics known to

Continued

TREATMENT

Miscellaneous Code Drugs
Continued

SODIUM BICARBONATE
Continued

produce hypochloremic alkalosis, and in those on salt restriction.
Possible side effects
GI disturbances, such as increased stomach acid secretion, gastric distention, abdominal cramps, anorexia, nausea, and vomiting; dizziness, convulsions; thirst; diminished respirations; renal calculi or crystals; with overdose, alkalosis, hypernatremia, hyperosmolarity
Special Considerations
• May be added to I.V. solution,

unless solution contains epinephrine or norepinephrine.
• Do not infuse through I.V. line containing calcium, or the drug will precipitate.
• Obtain arterial blood gas (ABG) and serum electrolyte measurements during administration and report changes.
• Too rapid administration of sodium bicarbonate may cause severe alkalosis which may be accompanied by hyperirritability or tetany.
• Prolonged sodium bicarbonate therapy isn't recommended because of the high risk of metabolic alkalosis or sodium overload.

TREATMENT

Adrenergics

DOPAMINE HYDROCHLORIDE
Intropin*

Indications
• Cardiogenic shock

*Also available in Canada.

• Hypovolemic shock associated with trauma, septicemia, open heart surgery, renal failure, congestive heart failure

Continued

Adrenergics
Continued

DOPAMINE HYDROCHLO-
RIDE
Intropin*
Continued

Dosage
Adults
I.V. infusion: 2 to 5 mcg/kg/
min. Severely ill patients may
receive up to 50 mcg/kg/min.
Children
I.V. infusion: 2 to 5 mcg/kg/
min. May increase to no more
than 20 mcg/kg/min.

Contraindications
- Uncorrected tachyarrhyth-
mias
- Pheochromocytoma
- Ventricular fibrillation
- With caution if patient has
occlusive vascular disease,
cold injuries, diabetic endar-
teritis, arterial embolism
- With caution in pregnant females
- With caution if patient is receiving MAO inhibitors

Possible side effects
Cardiac dysrhythmias, palpitations, widening of QRS intervals, headache, dizziness,
pallor, sweating, nausea,
vomiting, restlessness, tremors, weakness, respiratory
difficulty, anginal-type pain,
hypotension

Special considerations
- Monitor patient's blood
pressure every 5 minutes, his
cardiac conduction continuously, and his urine output
hourly. Report any changes
to doctor.
- Check infusion site frequently
for extravasation. If extravasation occurs, doctor may infiltrate
site with 5 to 10 mg of phentolamine with 10 to 15 ml normal
saline solution.
- Use infusion pump.
- Mix drug with I.V. solution
just before administration.
- Don't mix dopamine with
other drugs.
- If drug is stopped, watch
closely for sudden drop in
blood pressure.
- Dopamine solutions deterio-
rate after 24 hours. Discard
at that time or earlier if solution is discolored.
- Do not give alkaline drugs
through I.V. line containing
dopamine.

Continued

Adrenergics
Continued

DOBUTAMINE
Dobutrex

Dose and route
For refractory congestive heart failure: 2.5 to 10 mcg/kg/min. as I.V. infusion. Increase rate to 40 mcg/kg/min.

Interactions
Beta-adrenergic blockers: may decrease dobutamine's effectiveness. Use together cautiously.

Possible side effects
Tachycardia, hypertension, premature ventricular contractions

Special considerations
• Monitor EKG, blood pressure, PCWP, and cardiac output continuously. Also monitor urinary output.

• Incompatible with alkaline solutions. Oxidation of drug may slightly discolor admixtures. This does not indicate a significant loss of potency. I.V. solutions remain stable for 24 hours.

• A unique agent. Increases contractility of failing heart without inducing marked tachycardia, except at high doses.

• Often used with nitroprusside for additive effects.

• Infusions of up to 72 hours produce no more adverse effects than shorter infusions.

• Dobutamine is a chemical modification of isoproterenol.

EPINEPHRINE HYDRO-CHLORIDE
Adrenalin*

Indications
• Cardiac and circulatory failure
• Hypotensive states
• Allergic reactions
• Angioneurotic edema
• Status asthmaticus

Dosage
Adults
I.M. or subcutaneously: 0.1 to 0.5 ml in 1% solution, injected slowly. May dilute to 10 ml with normal saline solution.
Intracardiac: 1 ml of 1% solution. May repeat.

Children
I.V. or intracardiac: 0.1 ml/kg of 1% solution, up to a maximum of 3 ml. May dilute to 10

Continued

TREATMENT

Adrenergics
Continued

EPINEPHRINE HYDRO-
CHLORIDE
Adrenalin*
Continued

ml with saline solution. May
repeat every 5 minutes.
Contraindications
• Shock other than anaphy-
lactic, ventricular fibrillation,
and narrow angle glaucoma
• With caution in elderly patient who has angina, hypertension, or hyperthyroidism
Possible side effects
Cerebral hemorrhage, cardiac
dysrhythmias, palpitations,
widened pulse pressure, precordial pain, headache, nervousness, vertigo, tremor,
sweating, nausea, weakness,
dizziness, tachycardia, hyperglycemia, EKG changes
Special considerations
• Don't mix with alkaline solutions. Use dextrose 5% in
water, normal saline solution,
or a combination of dextrose
5% in water and saline solution. Mix just before use.
• Epinephrine is rapidly de-
stroyed by oxidizing agents,
such as iodine, chromates,
nitrates, nitrites, oxygen, and

salts of easily reducible met-
als, such as iron.
• Epinephrine solutions dete-
riorate after 24 hours. Discard after that time or before
if solution is discolored or
contains precipitate. Keep solution in light-resistant container, and don't remove
before use.
• Do not expose drug to light,
heat, or air.
• If given intravenously, take
baseline blood pressure and
pulse before initiation of therapy. Monitor closely every
minute until desired effect is
reached, then every 2 minutes until patient stabilizes.
After patient stabilizes, monitor blood pressure every 15
minutes.
• If patient experiences sharp
increase in blood pressure,
administer rapid-acting vasodilators, as ordered.

ISOPROTERENOL HYDRO-
CHLORIDE
Isuprel*

Indications
• Cardiac standstill

Continued

Adrenergics
Continued

ISOPROTERENOL HYDRO-
CHLORIDE
Isuprel*
Continued

- Carotid sinus syndromes
- Bradycardia
- AV heart block

Dosage
Adults
I.V. infusion: 2 mg in 500 ml
of 5% dextrose in water. Adjust infusion according to
heart rate.
I.V. bolus: 0.02 to 0.06 mg,
then 0.01 to 0.2 mg as necessary.
I.M.: 0.2 mg initially, then 0.2
to 1 mg as necessary.
Intracardiac: 0.02 mg (in extreme cases).
Children
I.V. infusion: 1 mg in 100 ml
of 5% dextrose in water. Give
at 0.1 to 0.5 mcg/kg/min. Adjust rate to patient's response.
Contraindications
- Tachycardia
- Preexisting dysrhythmias
- With caution if patient has
coronary insufficiency, diabetes, hyperthyroidism

*Also available in Canada

Possible side effects
Tachycardia, palpitations,
bronchial edema, flushing,
headache, cardiac dysrhythmias, chest pain, tremors,
anxiety, fatigue, nausea and
vomiting, swelling of parotid
glands
Special considerations
- Correct volume deficit before
administering vasopressors.
- Closely monitor patient's
heart rate and rhythm, blood
pressure, CVP, EKG, ABGs,
and urinary output. If heart
rate exceeds 110 bpm, slow
down or discontinue infusion.
A heart rate over 130 bpm
may trigger ventricular dysrhythmias.
- If anginal pain occurs, stop
drug immediately.
- Use an infusion pump,
when administering I.V.
- This drug may cause slight
rise in systolic pressure and
drop in diastolic pressure.

METARAMINOL BITARTRATE
Aramine*

Indications
- To prevent and treat hypo-
Continued

TREATMENT

Adrenergics
Continued

METARAMINOL BITARTRATE
Aramine*
Continued

tension due to shock
Dosage
Adults
I.M. or S.C.: 2 to 10 mg.
I.V. bolus: 0.5 to 5 mg followed by I.V. infusion.
I.V. infusion: 15 to 100 mg in 500 ml 5% dextrose in water or normal saline solution, adjust rate to maintain blood pressure at desired level.
Children
I.V. bolus: 0.01 mg/kg.
I.V. infusion: 1 mg in 25 ml 5% dextrose in water. Adjust rate to maintain adequate blood pressure.
I.M.: 0.1 mg/kg, as needed.
Contraindications
• Pulmonary edema; cardiac arrest; during anesthesia with cyclopropane and halogenated hydrocarbons
• With caution in patients with heart disease, hypertension, thyroid disease, diabetes, cirrhosis, or malaria, or with pa-
*Also available in Canada

tients receiving digitalis
Possible side effects
Cerebral hemorrhage, cardiac dysrhythmias, precordial pain, headache, vertigo, tremor, hyper/hypotension, nervousness, sweating, nausea, pallor, respiratory difficulty, hyperglycemia, decreased urinary output
Special considerations
• Correct volume deficit before administering vasopressors.
• Obtain baseline blood pressure reading. Then, monitor every 15 minutes during administration.
• Drug may cause hyperglycemia. Closely monitor diabetic patient.
• When administering by I.V. infusion, use an infusion pump. Avoid extravasation.
• When discontinuing drug, gradually slow infusion rate.
• Keep solution in light-resistant container, away from heat. Do not mix with other drugs.
• Keep atropine on hand to treat reflux bradycardia, phentolamine to decrease vasopressor effects, and propranolol to treat dysrhythmias.

Continued

Adrenergics
Continued

NOREPINEPHRINE, FOR-
MERLY CALLED LEVARTE-
RENOL BITARTRATE

Levophed*
Indications
• To treat acute hypotensive
states or MI
Dosage
Adults
I.V. infusion: initially 8 to 12
mcg/min. Then adjust to
maintain blood pressure at
desired level.
Contraindications
• Peripheral vascular thrombosis
• Hypoxia
• Pregnancy
• Hypotension
• With caution if patient has
heart disease or obstruction
of urinary tract, hypertension,
or hyperthyroidism
• Do not administer with cyclopropane and halothane anesthesia
• With caution if patient is receiving MAO inhibitors or tricyclic antidepressants
Possible side effects
Cerebral hemorrhage, cardiac

*Also available in Canada

dysrhythmias, precordial pain,
excess CNS stimulation, headache, nervousness, tremors, in-
somnia, sweating, nausea, pallor,
Special considerations
• Take a baseline blood pressure reading before administration.
• Check blood pressure every 2 minutes during and after administration to ensure
that desired drug level is
maintained.
• Administer via large vein,
using infusion pump. Try to
avoid extravasation. If it occurs, stop infusion, and infiltrate area with 5 to 10 mg
phentolamine and 10 to 15 ml
normal saline solution.
• When discontinuing therapy, slow infusion rate gradually. Monitor vital signs.
• Administer in dextrose and
saline solution; saline solution
alone is not recommended.
• Incompatible with whole
blood and plasma. Administer
separately.
• Use atropine to treat reflex
bradycardia and propranolol
to treat dysrhythmias.

TREATMENT

Antiarrhythmics

AMIODARONE HYDRO-CHLORIDE†

Cordarone
Dose and route
Adults
Loading dose is 5 to 10 mg/kg by I.V. infusion via central line, followed by I.V. infusion of 10 mg/kg per day for 3 to 5 days. Maintenance dose: 200 to 600 mg P.O. daily.
Interactions
None significant
Side effects
Peripheral neuropathy and extrapyramidal symptoms, headache, bradycardia, hypotension, corneal microdeposits, hypo- and hyperthyroidism, altered liver enzymes, hepatic dysfunction, pneumonitis, photosensitivity, blue-gray skin pigmentation, muscle weakness
Special considerations
• Use cautiously in patients with preexisting bradycardia or sinus node disease, conduction disturbances, severely depressed ventricular function, and marked cardiomegaly.
• Amiodarone is often effective for treatment of dysrhythmias resistant to other drug therapy. However, large incidence of side effects limits its use.

BRETYLIUM

Bretylol
Dose and route
5 to 10 mg/kg I.V. q 15 to 30 minutes to maximum of 30 mg/kg followed by maintenance dose of 5 to 10 mg/kg q 6 to 8 hours I.V. or I.M.
Interactions
None significant.
Side effects
Severe orthostatic hypotension and syncope, bradycardia, vertigo, dizziness
Special considerations
• Monitor blood pressure, heart rate, and rhythm frequently. Notify doctor immediately of significant changes. Keep patient supine until he develops tolerance to hypotension.
• Give I.V. injections for ventricular fibrillation as rapidly as possible; do not dilute. Rotate I.M. injection sites to prevent tissue damage, and don't exceed 5-ml volume in any one site.

Continued

TREATMENT

Antiarrhythmics
Continued

DISOPYRAMIDE

Rythmodan*
Dose and route
4 mg/kg P.O. followed by maintenance dose of 100 to 200 mg q 6 hours.
Interactions
Ethotoin, mephenytoin, phenytoin, rifampin: decreased disopyramide blood levels.
Side effects
Anticholinergic effects, blurred vision, dry mouth, urinary retention, hypotension, heart block
Special considerations
• Check apical pulse before administering drug. Notify doctor of change in pulse.
• Discontinue if heart block develops, if QRS complex widens by more than 25%, or if QT interval lengthens by more than 25%.

LIDOCAINE

Lido Pen Auto-Injector, Xylocaine*

Dose and route
1 to 1.5 mg/kg I.V. bolus. Repeat q 3 to 5 minutes. Don't exceed 300 mg total bolus during 1-hour period. Follow with maintenance infusion of 1 to 4 mg/min.
Interactions
Procainamide: increased neurologic side effects
Beta-adrenergic blockers, cimetidine: increased pharmacologic effect of lidocaine
Succinylcholine: increased neuromuscular blocking effects
Side effects
Confusion, stupor, restlessness, light-headedness, convulsions, hypotension, tinnitus, blurred vision
Special considerations
• Contraindicated in complete or second-degree heart block. Use of lidocaine with epinephrine to treat dysrhythmias contraindicated. Use a reduced dose in elderly patients, those with CHF, renal or hepatic disease, or patients who weigh less than 50 kg.

Continued

TREATMENT

Unmarked trade names available in the United States only.
*Available in both the United States and in Canada.
†Investigational drug

Antiarrhythmics
Continued

LIDOCAINE
Continued

• In severely ill patients, convulsions may be first toxic sign.
• If toxic signs occur, stop drug at once and notify doctor. Give oxygen via nasal cannula, if not contraindicated. Keep oxygen and CPR equipment handy.
• During infusion, remain with patient and check cardiac monitor. Use an infusion pump or a microdrip system for monitoring infusion precisely. Never exceed an infusion rate of 4 mg/min. A bolus dose not followed by infusion will have a short-lived effect.
• Monitor patient's blood pressure, serum electrolytes, BUN, and creatinine. Tell doctor promptly if problems occur.

PHENYTOIN

Dilantin*

Dose and route
250 mg I.V. over 5 minutes until dysrhythmias subside (up to maximum dose of 1 g), or 1 g P.O. over 4 hours. Followed by maintenance dose of 200 to 400 mg I.V. or P.O. daily.
Interactions
Alcohol, barbiturates, folic acid, loxapine: monitor for decreased phenytoin activity.
Oral anticoagulants, antihistamines, chloramphenicol, diazepam, diazoxide, disulfiram, isoniazide, phenylbutazone, salicylates, sulfonamides, cimetidine, trimethoprim, valproic acid: monitor for increased phenytoin activity.
Corticosteroids/Levodopa: may need higher dose
Primidone: increased primidone toxicity.
Quinidine: decreased pharmacologic action.
Theophyllines: decreased pharmacologic effects of both drugs.
Side effects
Ataxia, nystagmus, lethargy,
Continued

TREATMENT

Antiarrhythmics
Continued

PHENYTOIN
Dilantin*
Continued

blood dyscrasias, severe hypotension, and vascular collapse (if given too rapidly by I.V.)
Special considerations
• Watch patients on phenytoin and other antiarrhythmics for signs of additive cardiac depression. Phenytoin can be diluted in normal saline solution and infused without precipitation. Infusions should not take longer than 1 hour. Don't mix with 5% dextrose I.V. fluids, as crystallization will occur. Flush I.V. line with saline solution before and after administration. Give drug by slow I.V. push, not to exceed 50 mg/min. in adults.
• Monitor blood pressure and EKG. Notify doctor if side effects occur.
• Blood levels greater than 20 mcg/ml may be toxic. The difference between therapeutic and toxic levels of phenytoin in blood is very slight. If toxic symptoms occur, draw blood to determine drug level.

PROCAINAMIDE

Procan, ProcanSR, Pronestyl*, Pronestyl-SR, Sub-Quin
Dose and route
100 mg q 5 minutes by slow I.V. push to maximum of 1 g (or 1 to 1.25 g P.O.), followed by I.V. infusion of 2 to 6 mg/minute. Maintenance P.O. dose is 500 mg to 1 g q 4 to 6 hours.
Interactions
None significant
Side effects
Lupus-like syndrome, blood dyscrasias, hypotension, nausea, vomiting, maculopapular rash
Special considerations
• Contraindicated in patients with hypersensitivity to procaine and related drugs; with complete, second-, or third-degree heart block unassisted by electrical pacemaker; or with myasthenia gravis. Use with caution in congestive heart failure or other conduction disturbances, such as bundle branch block or cardiotonic glycoside intoxication, or with

Continued

TREATMENT

Antiarrhythmics
Continued

PROCAINAMIDE
Continued

hepatic or renal insufficiency.
• Continuously observe patient. Use an infusion pump or a microdrip system and timer to monitor the infusion precisely. Monitor blood pressure and EKG continuously during I.V. administration. Watch for prolonged QT and QR intervals, heart block, or increased dysrhythmias. If these occur, withhold drug, obtain rhythm strip, and notify doctor immediately.
• Keep patient in supine position for I.V. administration.
• Patient with CHF has a lower volume of distribution and requires lower doses.
• After long-standing atrial fibrillation, restoration of normal rhythm may result in thromboembolism, due to dislodgement of thrombi from atrial wall. Anticoagulation usually advised before restoration of normal sinus rhythm.
• Urge patient compliance.

PROPRANOLOL HYDRO-CHLORIDE

Inderal*
Dose and route
1 to 5 mg I.V. infused slowly, not to exceed 1 mg/minute. Oral maintenance dose is 10 to 80 mg t.i.d. or q.i.d.
Interactions
Prazosin: increased hypotension
Lidocaine: increased pharmacologic effect; monitor for toxicity
Theophyllines: decreased therapeutic effect
Barbiturates, indomethacin, rifampin, thyroid hormones: decreased pharmacologic effect of propranolol
Chlorpromazine, cimetidine, oral contraceptives: increased pharmacologic effect of propranolol
Side effects
Heart block, bradycardia, hypotension, heart failure, asthma, fatigue
Special considerations
• Check apical pulse and blood pressure before giving drug. If you detect extremes in

Continued

TREATMENT

Antiarrhythmics
Continued

pulse rate, withhold drug and notify doctor. Monitor patient daily for weight gain and peripheral edema. Auscultate for rales and S_3 or S_4. If these develop, notify doctor. Always withdraw drug slowly. Abrupt withdrawal might precipitate MI or aggravate angina, thyrotoxicosis, or pheochromocytoma. Before any surgery, notify anesthesiologist that patient is receiving drug.

Double-check dose and route. (I.V. doses much smaller than P.O.).

QUINIDINE (all salts)

Biquin Durules**, Duraquin, Quinaglute Dura-Tabs*, Quinate**, Cardioquin*, CinQuin, Quine, Quinidex Extentabs, Quinora, SK-Quinidine Sulfate
Dose and route
200 to 400 mg P.O. (quinidine sulfate or equivalent base) q 4 to 6 hours
Interactions
Acetazolamide, antacids, sodium bicarbonate: increased quinidine blood levels due to alkaline urine
Barbiturates, phenytoin, rifampin: antagonized quinidine activity
Verapamil: don't use together in cardiomyopathy. May cause hypotension.
Digoxin: increased toxicity
Oral anticoagulants: increased pharmacologic effect. Monitor prothrombin time.
Side effects
Diarrhea, nausea, vomiting, cinchonism, thrombocytopenia, hypertension, heart block, EKG changes
Special considerations
• Use with caution in digitalized patients. Monitor digitalis levels. GI side effects, especially diarrhea, indicate toxicity. Notify doctor if these occur. GI symptoms may be decreased by giving with meals.
• Instruct patient to notify doctor if skin rash, fever, unusual bleeding, bruising, tinnitus, or visual disturbance occurs.

Continued

TREATMENT

Unmarked trade names available in the United States only.
*Available in both the United States and in Canada.
**Available in Canada only.

Antiarrhythmics
Continued

VERAPAMIL

Calan, Isoptin*
Dose and route
5 to 10 mg I.V. bolus over 2 to 3 minutes followed by a maintenance infusion
Interactions
Quinidine: don't use together in cardiomyopathy; may cause hypotension
Digoxin: increased blood levels
Beta-adrenergic blockers: increased risk of congestive heart failure
Side effects
Hypotension, heart failure, heart block, asystole
Special considerations
• Patient with severely compromised cardiac function or patient receiving beta blockers should receive lower doses of verapamil. Monitor these patients closely.
• In older patients, give I.V. doses over at least 3 minutes to minimize the risk of adverse effects.
• Notify doctor if signs of congestive heart failure occur.

TOCAINIDE HYDROCHLORIDE

Tonocard
Dose and route
400 mg P.O. every 8 hours. Dosage range 1200 to 1800 mg/day in 3 equally divided doses.
Interactions
None significant
Side effects
CNS: lightheadedness, dizziness, tremor, nervousness, confusion, altered mood, ataxia, visual disturbances, paresthesia
GI: nausea, anorexia, vomiting, diarrhea
CV: increased ventricular arrhythmia, progression of CHF
Other: skin rash, sweating
Special considerations
• Contraindicated in patients with second- or third-degree AV block in the absence of an artificial ventricular pacemaker.
• Use cautiously in patients with known heart failure.
• Patients who are successful with this dosing may be tried

TREATMENT

Antiarrhythmics
Continued

TOCAINIDE HYDROCHLO-
RIDE
Continued

on a twice-daily dose regimen
with careful monitoring.
• Administer reduced dosage
in patients with renal or hepatic
problems
• Patients who respond to lidocaine usually respond to
tocainide.

• Tremor indicates approach
of maximum dose.
• Although side effects occur
in up to 70% of all patients,
they're usually considered
mild or transient.
• May administer oral maintenance dose with meals.
• Tocainide has little or no
adverse effect on the EKG
heart rate or blood pressure.

Antianginals

DILTIAZEM

Cardizem
Dose and route
30 to 60 mg P.O. q.i.d.
Interactions
Beta-adrenergic blockers: in-
creased risk of CHF
Side effects
Headache, fatigue, drowsi-
ness, edema, dysrhythmias,
nausea, skin rash
Special considerations
If nitrate therapy is prescribed
during titration of diltiazem
dosage, urge patient to con-

tinue compliance. Sublingual
nitroglycerin may be taken
when anginal symptoms are
acute.

ISOSORBIDE DINITRATE

Isordil*, Sorbitrate
Dose and route
2.5 to 10 mg q 2 to 3 hours
p.r.n. sublingual or chewable
form; 5 to 30 mg P.O. q.i.d.
for prophylaxis

Continued

TREATMENT

Antianginals
Continued

ISOSORBIDE DINITRATE
Continued

Interactions
Ergot alkaloids: increased
toxic effects
Side effects
Throbbing headache, dizziness, orthostatic hypotension,
tachycardia, palpitations, an-
kle edema, flushing
Special considerations
• Monitor blood pressure and
intensity and duration of response to drug. Additional
dose may be taken before
anticipated stress or at bed-
time if angina is nocturnal.
Warn patient not to confuse
sublingual with oral form. Advise him to avoid alcohol.
• Teach patient to take sublingual tablet at first sign of attack.
He should wet the tablet with
saliva, place it under the tongue
until completely absorbed, and
sit down and rest. Dose may be
repeated every 10 to 15 minutes for a maximum of three
doses. If no relief, patient
should call doctor immediately.

NADOLOL

Corgard*
Dose and route
80 to 240 mg P.O. once daily
Interactions
Prazosin: increased hypoten-
sion
Lidocaine: increased blood
levels
Theophyllines: decreased
therapeutic effect
Indomethacin: decreased
therapeutic effect of nadolol
Side effects
Bradycardia, hypotension,
CHF, airway resistance
Special considerations
• Always check apical pulse
before giving drug. If slower
than 60 beats/minute, hold drug
and call doctor.
• Monitor blood pressure. If
patient develops hypotension,
give vasopressor, as ordered.
• Don't discontinue abruptly.
• This drug masks signs of
shock and hypoglycemia.
• May be given without regard
to meals.

Continued

TREATMENT

Antianginals
Continued

NIFEDIPINE

Adalat**, Procardia
Dose and route
10 to 30 mg P.O. q.i.d.
Interactions
Beta-adrenergic blockers: increased risk of congestive heart failure
Side effects
Dizziness, light-headedness, flushing, headache, nausea, heartburn
Special considerations
• Monitor blood pressure regularly.
• Patient may briefly develop anginal exacerbation when beginning drug therapy or at times of dosage increase. Reassure him that this symptom is temporary.
• If patient is on nitrate therapy while drug dosage is being titrated, urge him to continue his compliance. Sublingual nitroglycerin may be taken as needed when anginal symptoms are acute.

• Instruct patient to swallow capsule whole without breaking, crushing, or chewing.

NITROGLYCERIN

Nitro-Bid, Nitrol*
Dose and route
0.15 to 0.6 mg sublingually q 5 minutes p.r.n.; 1 to 2 inches ointment q 4 hours; 5 to 10 mg transdermal patch applied q 24 hours
Interactions
Ergot alkaloids: increased toxic effects
Side effects
Headache, dizziness, orthostatic hypotension, tachycardia, flushing, palpitations
Special considerations
• Monitor blood pressure and intensity and duration of response to drug.
• Advise patient to avoid alcohol.
• Only sublingual form should be used in acute attack. Teach

TREATMENT

Continued

Antianginals
Continued

NITROGLYCERIN
Continued

patient to take tablet at first
sign of attack. If no relief, he
should call doctor or go to
emergency department.
• To apply ointment, spread
in uniformly thin layer on any
nonhairy area. Do not rub in.
Cover with plastic film to aid
absorption and to protect
clothing.
• Transdermal dosage forms
can be applied to any hair-
less part of the skin except
distal parts of the arms or
legs.

VERAPAMIL

Calan, Isoptin*
Dose and route
240 to 480 mg P.O. daily in
divided doses
Interactions
Beta-adrenergic blockers: in-
creased risk of CHF. Use to-
gether cautiously.
Digoxin: elevated blood level.
Monitor for toxicity.

Quinidine: don't use together
in cardiomyopathy.
Side effects
Hypotension, heart failure,
heart block, asystole.
Special considerations
• Notify doctor if signs of
CHF occur.
• If patient is kept on nitrate
therapy while dosage of verapamil is being titrated, urge
him to comply.
• Sublingual nitroglycerin
may be taken when anginal
symptoms are acute.

PROPRANOLOL HYDRO-
CHLORIDE

Inderal*, Inderal LA*
Dose and route
80 to 160 mg P.O. daily in
single dose (sustained-action
capsule) or divided doses
Interactions
Prazosin: increased hypotension
Lidocaine: increased blood
levels; monitor for toxicity
Theophyllines: decreased
therapeutic effect

Continued

Unmarked trade names available in the United States only.
*Available in both the United States and Canada.
**Available only in Canada.

Antianginals
Continued

PROPRANOLOL HYDRO-
CHLORIDE
Continued

---

*Barbiturates, indomethacin,
rifampin, thyroid hormones:*
decreased pharmacologic effect of propranolol
*Chlorpromazine, cimetidine,
oral contraceptives:* increased
pharmacologic effect of propranolol
Side effects
Fatigue, bradycardia, hypotension, CHF, airway resistance
Special considerations
• Contraindicated in asthma
or allergic rhinitis; during ethyl
ether anesthesia; in sinus
bradycardia and in heart
block greater than first de-

gree; in cardiogenic shock; in
right ventricular failure secondary to pulmonary hypertension. Use with caution in
patients with CHF, diabetes
mellitus, or respiratory disease.
• Always check patient's apical pulse rate before giving
this drug. If you detect extremes in pulse rates, hold
medication and call the doctor immediately. If patient develops hypotension, monitor
blood pressure frequently.
• Don't discontinue abruptly.
• This drug masks common
signs of shock and hypoglycemia.
• Food may increase the absorption of propranolol. Give
consistently with meals.

TREATMENT

Highlighting Calcium Channel Blockers

You've probably cared for patients taking nifedipine (Procardia), diltiazem (Cardisem), or
verapamil (Calan). Or perhaps
you've seen verapamil I.V. given
in a cardiac emergency.

All these drugs are calcium
channel blockers that work
by:
• decreasing myocardial oxygen demand by reducing
myocardial contractility and
dilating peripheral arterioles
Continued

Highlighting Calcium Channel Blockers
Continued

TREATMENT

• improving myocardial perfusion by dilating coronary arteries
• reducing electrical excitation.

In the normal cell, calcium ions trigger a chemical reaction inside each myocardial cell, causing it to contract; but before this can happen, the cell must take in additional calcium ions from the extracellular space. It does this by changing its membrane, opening channels to receive outside calcium ions.

Calcium channel blockers close off some channels, limiting calcium's passage into the cell during depolarization so that fewer calcium ions are present to trigger the reaction. The muscle cell contracts, but not as forcefully.

Uses
Nifedipine, diltiazem, and oral verapamil all treat typical and variant (Prinzmetal's) angina. They also reduce coronary artery spasms in patients with Prinzmetal's angina.

Verapamil I.V. inhibits calcium influx into myocardial conduction fibers of sinoatrial and atrioventricular nodes. Because of this, it's used to treat supraventricular tachy-dysrhythmias, such as atrial fibrillation, atrial flutter, and paroxysmal supraventricular tachycardia. Diltiazem has similar, but less extensive, electrophysiologic effects. So far, the Food and Drug Administration hasn't approved it for treating supraventricular tachycardia dysrhythmias.

Nursing considerations
Be alert for:
• hypotension, especially if your patient's also taking antihypertensive drugs
• signs and symptoms of congestive heart failure, especially if your patient's also taking a beta-blocker
• bradycardia, heart blocks, and sinus arrest when verapamil I.V. is given (always connect him to a cardiac monitor)
• increased severity of anginal pain until the drug reaches therapeutic levels when nifedipine is given
• signs and symptoms of digitalis toxicity if your patient's also taking digoxin.

Calcium Channel Blockers

ALL CALCIUM CHANNEL
BLOCKERS: DILTIAZEM, NI-
FEDIPINE, VERAPAMIL

Interacting drug
• Beta blockers
• Disopyramide
Possible effect
Heart block from negative
inotropic effect of both
agents. *Note:* This interaction
is somewhat more significant
with verapamil.
Heart block from inhibition of
AV conduction by both drugs.
Note: This interaction is
somewhat more significant
with verapamil.
Nursing considerations
• Observe the patient for signs
and symptoms of congestive
heart failure. Teach him to recognize and report these signs
and symptoms.
• Check for breathing problems
and light-headedness.
• Instruct the patient to count
his pulse rate and to report an
abnormally slow rate (less than
50 beats/minute or as specified
by the doctor).
• Tell him to take the drugs only
in the prescribed dosages and

to consult a doctor before discontinuing the drugs, taking additional medications, or drinking
alcoholic beverages.
• Follow the same guidelines
listed on page 124.
Interacting drug
• Antihypertensives
• Digoxin
Possible effect
Additive hypotension. *Note:*
This interaction is somewhat
more significant with nifedipine.
Digitalis toxicity from increased
plasma digoxin levels. *Note:*
This interaction is somewhat
more significant with verapamil.
Nursing considerations
• Periodically check blood
pressure and pulse while the
patient is lying down, sitting,
and standing.
• Advise him to sit and stand
slowly to avoid dizziness.
• Observe the patient for signs
and symptoms of digitalis toxicity: nausea and vomiting, anorexia, diarrhea, dysrhythmias,
and green- or yellow-tinted vision.
• Monitor plasma digoxin levels. Therapeutic levels range
from 0.7 to 2.0 ng/ml.

TREATMENT

Diuretics

AMILORIDE
Midamor*

5 to 10 mg P.O. daily
Interactions
Potassium preparations: may
result in hyperkalemia. Use
together cautiously.
Side effects
Headache, nausea, vomiting,
anorexia, diarrhea, impo-
tence, hyperkalemia
Special considerations
Discontinue immediately if
potassium level exceeds 6.5
mEq/liter. Warn patient to
avoid excessive ingestion of
potassium. Give amiloride
with or after meals.

CHLOROTHIAZIDE
Diurel*

500 mg to 2 g P.O. or I.V.
daily in 2 divided doses
Interactions
Cardiac glycosides: hypokalemia may increase digitalis
toxicity.
Lithium: may cause lithium
toxicity.
Oral hypoglycemics: hypogly-

cemic effect antagonized.
Side effects
Volume depletion and dehydration, hypokalemia, hyperuricemia, hyperglycemia, rash
Special considerations
Patients on digitalis have increased risk of digitalis toxicity. May use with potassium-
sparing diuretic to prevent potassium loss.
   Only injectable thiazide.
For I.V. use only.

CHLORTHALIDONE
Hygroten*

25 to 100 mg P.O. daily
Interactions
Cardiac glycosides: hypokale-
mia may increase digitalis
toxicity.
Lithium: may cause lithium
toxicity.
Oral hypoglycemics: hypogly-
cemic effect antagonized.
Side effects
Volume depletion and dehy-
dration, hypokalemia, hyper-
uricemia, hyperglycemia, rash
Special considerations
Watch for hypokalemia.

Unmarked trade names available in the United States only
*Also available in Canada

Continued

TREATMENT

Diuretics
Continued

FUROSEMIDE
Lasix*

40 to 160 mg P.O. or I.M. daily for maintenance therapy. 40 to over 200 mg I.V.
Interactions
Cardiac glycosides: hypokalemia may increase digitalis toxicity.
Aminoglycoside antibiotics: increased ototoxicity.
Side effects
Volume depletion and dehydration, hypokalemia, hyperuricemia, hyperglycemia, fluid and electrolyte imbalances
Special considerations
Potent loop diuretic; can lead to profound water and electrolyte depletion. Watch for hypokalemia. Give I.V. doses over 1 to 2 minutes. Give P.O. and I.M. preparations in a.m., second doses in early p.m.

HYDROCHLOROTHIAZIDE
Hydro Diurel*

25 to 100 mg P.O. daily at once or in divided doses

Interactions
Cardiac glycosides: hypokalemia may increase digitalis toxicity.
Lithium: may cause lithium toxicity.
Oral hypoglycemics: hypoglycemic effect antagonized.
Side effects
Volume depletion and dehydration, hypokalemia, hyperuricemia, hyperglycemia, rash
Special considerations
Consult with doctor and dietitian to provide high-potassium diet. Watch for hypokalemia.

METOLAZONE
Zaroxolyn*

2.5 to 10 mg P.O. daily
Interactions
Cardiac glycosides: hypokalemia may increase digitalis toxicity.
Lithium: may cause lithium toxicity.
Oral hypoglycemics: hypoglycemic effect antagonized.
Side effects
Volume depletion and dehydration, hypokalemia, hyperuricemia, hyperglycemia, rash
Continued

TREATMENT

Diuretics
Continued

METOLAZONE
Continued

Special considerations
Watch for signs of hypokalemia. Diet should include high-potassium foods. Give drug in a.m. The elderly are susceptible to diuresis.

SPIRONOLACTONE
Aldactone*

25 to 100 mg P.O. daily in divided doses
Interactions
Potassium preparations: may result in hyperkalemia. Use together cautiously.
Side effects
Hyperkalemia, gynecomastia in males, menstrual disturbances

Special considerations
Warn patient to avoid excessive ingestion of potassium-rich foods or potassium-containing salt substitutes. Give drug with meals. The elderly are susceptible to diuresis.

TRIAMTERENE
Dyrenium*

100 mg P.O. b.i.d.
Interactions
Potassium preparations: may result in hyperkalemia. Use together cautiously.
Side effects
Hyperkalemia, nausea, vomiting
Special considerations
Warn patient to avoid excessive ingestion of potassium. Give drug after meals.

Antihypertensives

ATENOLOL
Tenormin

50 to 100 mg P.O. daily as a single dose
Unmarked trade names available in the United States only.
*Also available in Canada

Interactions
Prazosin: increased hypotension
Lidocaine: increased blood levels of lidocaine
Indomethacin: decreased antihypertensive effect. Monitor
Continued

Antihypertensives
Continued

ATENOLOL
Continued

blood pressure and adjust dosage
Theophyllines: decreased therapeutic effect
Side effects
Bradycardia, hypotension, congestive heart failure
Special considerations
Always check patient's apical pulse before giving this drug; if slower than 60 beats/minute, hold drug and call doctor. Monitor blood pressure frequently.

Explain importance of taking drug, even when patient feels well. Tell him not to discontinue drug suddenly, but to call doctor if unpleasant side effects develop. Counsel patient to take drug at regular time each day.

CAPTOPRIL
Capoten*

25 to 50 mg P.O. t.i.d.
Interactions
None significant
Side effects
Leukopenia, hypotension,

loss of taste, proteinuria, renal failure, skin rash
Special considerations
Question patient about impaired taste sensation. Should be taken 1 hour before meals. Monitor blood pressure and pulse rate.

CLONIDINE HYDROCHLORIDE
Catapres*

0.2 to 0.8 mg P.O. daily in divided doses
Interactions
Tricyclic antidepressants: decreased antihypertensive effect
Side effects
Drowsiness, mouth dryness, constipation, orthostatic hypotension
Special considerations
Monitor blood pressure and pulse rate frequently. Dosage is usually adjusted to patient's blood pressure and tolerance. May be given to rapidly lower blood pressure in some hypertensive emergencies. Advise patient to avoid sudden position changes and take last dose just before retiring.

Continued

TREATMENT

Antihypertensives
Continued

DIAZOXIDE
Hyperstat*

300 mg I.V. bolus push, administered in 30 seconds or less into peripheral vein
Interactions
Thiazide diuretics: increased effects of diazoxide
Side effects
Sodium and water retention, orthostatic hypotension, nausea, vomiting, hyperglycemia, headaches
Special considerations
Monitor blood pressure frequently. Notify doctor immediately if severe hypotension develops. Keep norepinephrine available. Monitor intake and output. Weigh patient daily and report any increase. Watch diabetics for severe hyperglycemia or hyperosmolar nonketotic coma.

GUANABENZ ACETATE
Wytensin

4 to 8 mg P.O. b.i.d.
Interactions
CNS depressants: increased sedation

Side effects
Drowsiness, sedation, dizziness, weakness, mouth dryness
Special considerations
Advise patient to drive a car or operate machinery cautiously until CNS effects are known. Warn that tolerance to alcohol or CNS depressants may decrease.

GUANADREL SULFATE
Hylorel

20 to 75 mg P.O. daily in divided doses.
Interactions
MAO inhibitors, sympathomimetics, methylphenidate, phenothiazines, tricyclic antidepressants: decreased antihypertensive action
Side effects
Fatigue, dizziness, orthostatic hypotension
Special considerations
Monitor supine and standing blood pressure, especially during dosage adjustment. Tell outpatient to avoid strenuous exercise and hot showers. Inform patient that
Continued

TREATMENT

Antihypertensives
Continued

GUANADREL SULFATE
Hylorel *Continued*

orthostatic hypotension can
be minimized by avoiding
sudden position changes.

GUANETHIDINE SULFATE
Ismelin*

25 to 50 mg P.O. daily
Interactions
MAO inhibitors, sympathomimetics, methylphenidate, phenothiazines, tricyclic antidepressants: decreased antihypertensive action
Side effects
Dizziness, weakness, orthostatic hypotension, nasal stuffiness, diarrhea, edema, weight gain, inhibition of ejaculation
Special considerations
Tell outpatient to avoid strenuous exercise and warn that hot showers may cause hypotensive reaction. Inform patient that orthostatic hypotension can be minimized by rising slowly and avoiding sudden position changes. Give this drug with meals to increase absorption.

HYDRALAZINE HYDROCHLORIDE
Apresoline*

10 to 50 mg P.O. q.i.d.; 10 to 20 mg I.M. or I.V. q 4 hours. Switch to oral administration.
Interactions
None significant
Side effects
Sodium retention and weight gain, lupus erythematosus-like syndrome, headache, tachycardia, angina
Special considerations
Monitor patient's blood pressure and pulse rate frequently. Watch closely for signs of lupus erythematosus-like syndrome (sore throat, fever, muscle and joint aches, skin rash). Call doctor immediately if any of these develop. Give this drug with meals to increase absorption.
Continued

TREATMENT

Antihypertensives
Continued

TREATMENT

LABETALOL
Trandate, Normodyne

Adults: 100 mg P.O. b.i.d.
with or without a diuretic.
Dose may be increased to
200 mg b.i.d. after 2 days.
Further dose increases may
be made every 1 to 3 days
until optimum response is
reached. Usual maintenance
dose is 200 to 400 mg b.i.d.
*For severe hypertension and
hypertensive emergencies—*
Adults: Dilute 200 mg to 200 ml
with 5% dextrose in water. Infuse at 2 mg per minute until
satisfactory response is obtained. Then stop the infusion.
May repeat q 6 to 8 hours.
Interactions
*Insulin, hypoglycemic drugs
(oral);* can alter dosage re-
quirements in previously stabilized diabetics. Observe
patient carefully.
Side effects
Vivid dreams, fatigue, headache, *orthostatic hypotension
and dizziness,* peripheral vascular disease, nasal stuffiness, hypoglycemia without
tachycardia, nausea, vomiting, diarrhea, sexual dysfunction, urinary retention, rash,
increased airway resistance.
Special considerations
• Contraindicated in patients
with bronchial asthma.
• Use cautiously in congestive heart failure, chronic
bronchitis, emphysema, and
preexisting peripheral vascular disease.
• Monitor blood pressure frequently. If patient develops
severe hypotension, notify
doctor. He may prescribe a
vasopressor.
• Teach patient about his disease and therapy. Explain
why it's important to take this
drug exactly as prescribed,
even when he's feeling well.
Tell outpatient not to discontinue this drug suddenly; abrupt
discontinuation can exacerbate
angina and MI. Tell patient to
call doctor if unpleasant side effects develop.
• This drug masks common
signs of shock and hypoglycemia.

Unmarked trade names available in United States only.
*Also available in Canada.
**Available in Canada only.

Continued

Antihypertensives
Continued

LABETALOL
Continued

- Labetalol is a beta-adrenergic blocker that also has unique alpha-adrenergic blocking effects.
- Unlike other beta blockers, labetalol does not decrease heart rate or cardiac output.
- Dizziness, the most troublesome side effect, tends to occur in early stages of treatment, in patients also receiving diuretics, and in patients receiving higher dosages. Inform patient that this can be minimized by rising slowly and avoiding sudden position changes.
- Studies show that labetalol side effects seem less common and more transient than those of other beta blockers.

METHYLDOPA
Aldomet*
Dopamet**

500 mg to 2 g P.O. daily in divided doses; 500 mg to 1 g q 6 hours, diluted in dextrose 5% in water, given I.V. over 30 to 60 minutes.

Interactions
Lithium: increased toxicity. Lithium dose may have to be decreased.
Side effects
Sedation, decreased mental acuity, hemolytic anemia, edema and weight gain, orthostatic hypotension, mouth dryness
Special considerations
Weigh patient daily. Notify doctor of any weight increase. Inform patient that orthostatic hypotension can be minimized by rising slowly and avoiding sudden position changes.

METOPROLOL TARTRATE
Betaloc**
Lopressor

50 to 100 mg P.O. daily in 2 or 3 divided doses
Interactions
Prazosin: increased hypotension
Lidocaine: increased blood levels
Theophyllines: decreased therapeutic effect.

Continued

TREATMENT

Antihypertensives
Continued

METOPROLOL TARTRATE
Betaloc**
Lopressor
Continued

Barbiturates, indomethacin, rifampin, thyroid hormones: decreased effect of metoprolol
Chlorpromazine, cimetidine, oral contraceptives: increased effect of metoprolol
Side effects
Bradycardia, hypotension, CHF
Special considerations
Monitor blood pressure. If patient develops severe hypotension, notify doctor. Tell outpatient not to discontinue this drug suddenly. Instruct patient to call doctor if unpleasant side effects develop. Food may increase absorption. Give consistently with meals.

MINOXIDIL
Loniten*

10 to 40 mg P.O. daily
Interactions
None significant

Side effects
Edema, weight gain, hypertrichosis, tachycardia
Special considerations
About 80% of patients experience hypertrichosis within 6 weeks of beginning treatment. Suggest a depilatory or shaving, and assure patient that extra hair will disappear within 1 to 6 months of stopping minoxidil. Advise patient not to discontinue drug.

NADOLOL
Corgard*

80 to 240 mg P.O. once daily
Interactions
Prazosin: increased hypotension
Lidocaine: increased blood levels of lidocaine
Theophyllines: decreased therapeutic effect of theophyllines
Indomethacin: decreased therapeutic effect of nadolol
Side effects
Bradycardia, hypotension, congestive heart failure, increased airway resistance

Continued

Unmarked trade names available in the United States only.
*Available in both the United States and Canada.
**Available in Canada only.

Antihypertensives
Continued

NADOLOL
Corgard* Continued

Special considerations
Check patient's apical pulse before giving this drug. If slower than 60 beats/minute, hold drug and call doctor. Tell outpatient not to discontinue drug, but to call doctor if side effects develop. This drug masks common signs of shock and hypoglycemia. May be given without regard to meals.

NITROPRUSSIDE
Nipride*
Nitropres

Infuse intravenously at 0.5 to 10 mcg/kg/minute. Average dose is 3 mcg/kg/minute.
Interactions
None significant
Side effects
Headache, dizziness, restlessness, muscle twitching, diaphoresis, nausea, vomiting
Special considerations
Because of light sensitivity, wrap I.V. solution in foil. Fresh solution has faint brownish tint. Discard after

24 hours.

Obtain baseline vital signs before giving drug, and find out what parameters the doctor wants to achieve. Check blood pressure every 5 minutes at start of infusion and after every rate change. If severe hypotension occurs, turn off I.V. and notify doctor.

PINDOLOL
Visken*

10 to 20 mg P.O. b.i.d.
Interactions
Prazosin: increased hypotension
Theophyllines: decreased therapeutic effect
Indomethacin: decreased therapeutic effect of pindolol
Side effects
Fatigue, lethargy, congestive heart failure, hypotension, increased airway resistance, muscle and joint pain
Special considerations
Always check apical pulse rate before giving drug. If you detect extremes in pulse rates, hold drug and call doctor. Tell patient not to discon-

Continued

TREATMENT

Antihypertensives
Continued

PINDOLOL
Continued

---

tinue this drug suddenly. This drug masks common signs of shock and hypoglycemia.

PRAZOSIN HYDROCHLORIDE
Minipress*

---

3 to 20 mg P.O. daily in divided doses
Interactions
Beta-adrenergic blockers: increased hypotension
Side effects
Dizziness, "first-dose syncope," palpitations, nausea, orthostatic hypotension, mouth dryness
Special considerations
If first dose exceeds 1 mg, patient may develop severe syncope. Increase dose slowly.

PROPRANOLOL HYDRO-CHLORIDE
Inderal*, Inderal LA*

---

160 to 480 mg daily

Interactions
See propranolol hydrochloride on pages 122-23.
Side effects
See propranolol hydrochloride on pages 122-23.
Special considerations
See propranolol hydrochloride on pages 122-23.

TIMOLOL MALEATE
Blocadren

---

10 to 20 mg P.O. b.i.d.
Interactions
Prazosin: increased hypotension
Theophyllines: decreased therapeutic effect
Indomethacin: decreased therapeutic effect of pindolol
Side effects
Fatigue, hypotension, congestive heart failure, bradycardia
Special considerations
Always check apical pulse rate before giving drug. Tell patient not to discontinue drug suddenly; abrupt discontinuation can exacerbate angina. This drug masks common signs of shock and hypoglycemia.

Cardiac Glycosides

DIGITOXIN

Loading dose 1.2 to 1.6 mg I.V. or P.O. in divided doses over 24 hours; maintenance dose 0.1 mg daily.

DIGOXIN

Loading dose 0.5 to 1 mg I.V. or P.O. in divided doses over 24 hours; maintenance 0.125 mg to 0.5 mg I.V. or P.O. daily. Large doses often needed for dysrhythmias.

Interactions

Antacids, cholestyramine, colestipol, kaolin-pectin, metoclopramide: decreased absorption of cardiac glycosides

Amphotericin B, bumetanide, carbenicillin, ticarcillin, corticosteroids, and diuretics: hypokalemia may increase cardiac glycoside toxicity

Parenteral calcium, thiazides: hypercalcemia and hypomagnesemia may increase cardiac glycoside toxicity.

Thyroid hormones: decreased therapeutic effectiveness of cardiac glycosides

Phenylbutazone, phenobarbital, phenytoin, rifampin: decreased digitoxin levels

Quinidine, nifedipine, and verapamil: increased digoxin blood levels

Anticholinergics: increased digoxin absorption of oral tablets

Amiloride: altered digoxin excretion

Side effects

Yellow-green halos around visual images, blurred vision, anorexia, nausea, vomiting, diarrhea, fatigue, generalized muscle weakness, agitation, hallucinations, increased severity of congestive heart failure, dysrhythmias

Special considerations

Hypothyroid patients are very sensitive to glycosides; hyperthyroid patients may need larger doses.

Obtain baseline data (heart rate and rhythm, blood pressure, electrolytes) before giving first dose.

Take apical-radial pulse for a full minute. Record and report to doctor any significant changes (sudden increase or decrease in rate, pulse defi-

Continued

TREATMENT

Cardiac Glycosides
Continued

DIGOXIN
Continued

cit, irregular beats, and particularly regularization of a
previously irregular rhythm).
Check blood pressure and
obtain 12-lead EKG with
these changes. Excessive
slowing of pulse rate (60
beats/minute or less) may be
a sign of toxicity. Hold drug
and notify doctor.
   Observe eating pattern.
Ask patient about symptoms
of toxicity. Instruct patient
and responsible family mem-
ber about drug action, dosage regimen, how to take
pulse, reportable signs, and
follow-up plans.

Highlighting Streptokinase

If streptokinase is given to a patient with an acute myocardial
infarction, his chances of sur-
vival and recovery may improve. Here's why:
   Streptokinase is a throm-
bolytic, so it dissolves the clot
occluding the artery. This improves myocardial perfusion
and, if the drug's given within
3 to 4 hours of the onset of
the patient's chest pain, it limits the infarction's size.
   Administering streptokinase
directly into the occluded coronary artery, using angiography
in a cardiac catheterization
laboratory, is the most effective treatment. (You may also
give streptokinase by continuous I.V. for such disorders as
pulmonary emboli and deep-
vein thrombosis.)
   Remember these important
points about administering
streptokinase:
• Always establish a perfusion baseline of peripheral
pulses.
• Before infusion, double-
check all doses and infusion
rates with another nurse.
• Don't give intramuscular or
intravenous injections during
infusion or for 24 hours afterward.

Continued

TREATMENT

Highlighting Streptokinase
Continued

• Establish two I.V. lines before infusion. Use one for streptokinase, the second for any other drugs you need to give.
• Align and immobilize the affected limb.
• Inspect the infusion site hourly for signs of bleeding. After infusion, inspect the site every 15 minutes the first hour, every 30 minutes for 2 to 8 hours, then once per shift.
• Monitor and document the following every hour, before and after infusion: the patient's pulses and color, and the sensitivity of his affected and unaffected limbs.
• Keep a laboratory flow sheet so you can monitor the following during and after infusion: partial thromboplastin time, prothrombin time, hemoglobin, and hematocrit.
• Monitor carefully, for dysrhythmias, any patient receiving intracoronary streptokinase for lysis of coronary artery thrombi.
• Test all the patient's nasogastric aspirate and his stools and urine for blood, during and after infusion.
• Apply direct pressure to the infusion site for at least 30 minutes after the catheter's removed.
• Watch the patient for flushing, itching, urticaria, headaches and muscle aches, and nausea. These may indicate a mild allergic and febrile reaction.

Urokinase Vs Streptokinase

Urokinase is produced in low levels by the body and found in urine. Urokinase transforms the inactive protein plasminogen into its active form, plasmin, which causes fibrin to disintegrate and thrombi to dissolve. Systemically, it produces a lytic state in the blood that counteracts all clotting.

Although effective, urokinase is quite expensive. Streptokinase, a less costly protein obtained from streptococci, forms an activator complex that transforms plasminogen equally as well.

TREATMENT

Nursing Responses to Streptokinase Reactions

Streptokinase can produce adverse reactions ranging from mild discomfort to dangerous dysrhythmias. If you initiate treatment quickly, you can prevent small problems, such as mild fever, from becoming big ones, such as hemorrhage.

ADVERSE REACTION	NURSING RESPONSE
Mild fever	• Give acetaminophen. Avoid aspirin-containing products, which prolong clotting time.
Mild-to-severe allergic reactions (more likely with I.V. than intracoronary streptokinase)	• Monitor the patient closely. • Treat symptoms. • Administer corticosteroids, antihistamines, adrenergic agents, or life support, as ordered.
Dysrhythmias	• Obtain a baseline EKG. Continue EKG monitoring during and immediately after therapy. • Treat dysrhythmias, as ordered.
Hemorrhage	• Monitor vital signs and consciousness level. • Inspect the skin for subcutaneous bleeding. • Check laboratory results for decreasing hemoglobin or hematocrit levels. • Monitor for development of hematoma or hemorrhage. • Prepare to give aminocaproic acid (Amicar), if ordered, to increase clotting ability. • Prepare to transfuse blood or blood products, if ordered.

TREATMENT

Guide to Some Drugs That Affect the Cardiovascular System

CLASSIFICATION	POSSIBLE SIDE EFFECTS
Anticonvulsants diazepam (Valium*)	• Hypotension, bradycardia, cardiovascular collapse
phenytoin sodium (Dilantin*)	• Hypotension, ventricular fibrillation, nystagmus, ataxia, diplopia, blurred vision
Antidepressants amitriptyline hydrochloride (Elavil*) doxepin hydrochloride (Sinequan*)	• Orthostatic hypotension, tachycardia, EKG changes, hypertension
Antipsychotics chlorpromazine hydrochloride (Thorazine) thioridazine (Mellaril*)	• Orthostatic hypotension, tachycardia, dysrhythmias
Cerebral stimulants amphetamine sulfate (Benzedrine*)	• Tachycardia, palpitations, hypertension, hypotension
caffeine (Nodoz, Vivarin)	• Tachycardia
Cholinergics (parasympathomimetics) bethanechol chloride (Urecholine*)	• Bradycardia, hypotension, cardiac arrest, tachycardia

Continued

*Available in U.S. and Canada. **Available in Canada only. All other products (no symbol) available in U.S. only.

TREATMENT

Guide to Some Drugs That Affect the Cardiovascular System
Continued

CLASSIFICATION	POSSIBLE SIDE EFFECTS
Estrogens chlorotrianisene (Tace*) esterified estrogens (Amnestrogen, Climestrone**)	• Thrombophlebitis, thromboembolism, hypertension, edema, risk of cerebrovascular accident, pulmonary embolism, myocardial infarction
Nonnarcotic analgesics and antipyretics indomethacin (Indocid**, Indocin)	• Hypertension, edema
phenylbutazone (Butazolidin*)	• Hypertension, pericarditis, myocarditis, cardiac decompensation
Oral contraceptives estrogen with progestogen (Demulen*)	• Thromboembolism, thrombophlebitis, hypertension
Sedatives and hypnotics ethchlorvynol (Placidyl*) paraldehyde (Paral)	• Hypotension • By I.V. administration: pulmonary edema, hemorrhage, right-sided heart failure
Spasmolytics aminophylline (Aminophyllin)	• Sinus tachycardia, extrasystoles, flushing, hypotension

TREATMENT

*Available in U.S. and Canada. **Available in Canada only. All other products (no symbol) available in U.S. only.

Beta-Adrenergic Blockers: Highlighting Important Interaction

ALL BETA-ADRENERGIC
BLOCKERS: Atenolol, Labe-
talol, Metoprolol, Nadolol,
Pindolol, Propranolol, Timolol

Interacting drug
• All bronchodilators; for example, albuterol, aminophyl-
line, metaproterenol, terbuta-
line, and theophylline
Possible effect
Bronchospasm and wheezing
from antagonistic action of
beta blocker; reduced theophylline effectiveness from
antagonistic action of beta
blocker
Nursing considerations
• Check the patient's history
for asthma.
• Monitor him for signs and
symptoms of pulmonary disorders: wheezing, shortness
of breath, restlessness, increased pulse rate, thready
pulse, and dizziness.
• Instruct the patient to re-

port breathing problems and
warn him not to stop taking
the drug without consulting
the doctor.
• To minimize this interaction,
the doctor may order a car-
dioselective beta blocker,
such as atenolol or metoprolol.
• Monitor the patient for theophylline effectiveness.
• Monitor plasma theophylline
levels. Therapeutic levels
range from 10 to 20 mcg/ml.
If necessary, suggest that the
doctor increase the theophylline dosage.
• If theophylline dosage is increased during beta-adrenergic blocker therapy, make
sure theophylline dosage is
decreased again when beta
blocker dosage is decreased
or stopped.
• Assess the patient for
breathing problems.

Intraaortic Balloon Pump (IABP): Diastolic Augmentation

This graph demonstrates how the intraaortic balloon pump (IABP) augments diastolic pressure. The inflation-deflation cycle is synchronized with the R wave on the EKG. The R wave triggers deflation, which begins just before the central aortic upstroke. Inflation begins at the dicrotic notch in early diastole. Note that in an unassisted arterial pressure wave form, peak arterial pressure is during systole. When assisted by the IABP (below), peak arterial pressure is during diastole, enhancing coronary blood flow. Systolic pressure drops sharply when assisted, decreasing the left ventricle's work load and increasing cardiac output.

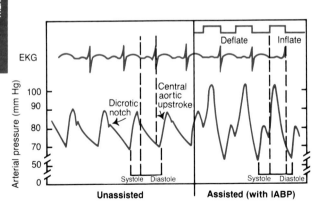

Intraaortic Balloon Catheter Placement

To insert a balloon catheter percutaneously, the doctor punctures the patient's femoral artery with an angiographic needle. He then makes an incision where the needle exits the skin and inserts a dilator to expand the vessel. Next, the doctor removes that dilator and replaces it with the percutaneous introducer dilator and sheath. Just before inserting the balloon catheter, the doctor removes the introducer dilator. He then feeds the balloon catheter into the sheath and through the femoral artery.

The balloon is tightly wound for insertion. Balloon size varies from patient to patient because the inflated balloon must never completely occlude the artery. Once in place, the balloon is unwound to facilitate inflation. Before removal, the balloon must be deflated.

Caring for the Patient on an Intraaortic Balloon Pump

To help manage the patient on an intra-aortic balloon pump, study the following list:
• Take your patient's baseline vital signs and neurologic signs before the procedure; then every 15 minutes afterward until he is stable; then once each hour.
• In addition, assess the following at least once an hour: your patient's cardiac rhythm, cardiac output, urinary output, pulmonary artery pressure (PAP), and the arterial pulse, temperature, and skin color of the leg with the insertion site.
• Assess pulmonary capillary wedge pressure (PCWP) every four hours, or as needed.

• Check the insertion site for signs of bleeding, inflammation, or infection.
• Inspect the balloon catheter regularly for signs of kinking or cracking. Make sure the catheter pump joint is connected securely.
• Check the EKG occasionally to make sure the R wave remains large enough to trigger the balloon pump. Eliminate any artifacts. Also, examine the arterial pressure wave and adjust inflation or deflation timing, if necessary.
• Draw arterial blood samples for clotting studies, platelet counts, and arterial blood gas values, as the doctor orders.
• Turn your patient by logrolling.

IABP Complications

• wound sepsis (The doctor will probably order a broad spectrum antibiotic to minimize infection risk. Of course, maintaining strict aseptic technique during the insertion procedure and subsequent dressing changes also helps prevent infection.)
• hematologic complications, including platelet depression. Be alert for hematoma or bleeding at the insertion site.

• arterial complications related to preexisting peripheral vascular disease or vascular trauma during insertion (for example, aortic trauma or dissection).
• thromboembolic complications, such as embolization or thrombi, which commonly occur in patients with peripheral vascular disease.

Special Note

If the balloon pump fails, notify the doctor and take steps to keep the balloon in motion while the pump is being fixed or another is being located. For example, some pumps have a flutter feature, which, when used, keeps the balloon moving slightly. If this feature isn't operating or isn't available, detach the connector tubing from the pump and connect a syringe to the tub-

ing. Every 5 minutes, rapidly inflate and deflate the balloon with small amounts of air. By keeping the balloon in motion, you prevent blood from clotting in the folds of the balloon membrane. *Caution:* Don't do this flutter procedure if the console indicates the balloon is broken or leaking, or if you see blood in the balloon catheter. Call the doctor at once.

TREATMENT

Troubleshooting Intraaortic Balloon Pump (IABP) Therapy

BALLOON IS INFLATING TOO FREQUENTLY OR ERRATICALLY

Possible cause
• Patient has a pacemaker
Solution
• Manipulate EKG leads so you get a dominant R wave and minimized pacemaker spike.
• Set the pacemaker on the lowest threshold level.
• Switch to arterial pressure triggering.
Possible cause
• Patient has multiple atrial dysrhythmias
Solution
• Treat per doctor's orders.
• Set timing to the most common RR interval (preferably short) while treating dysrhythmias.
Possible cause
• Artifact on EKG tracing caused by the equipment
Solution
• Eliminate artifact or switch to arterial pressure triggering.

AUGMENTATION CURVE (pressure curve caused by balloon inflation) IS ABSENT OR TOO SMALL

Possible cause
• Pump turned off
• No gas in balloon
Solution
• Turn on the pump.
• Check gas supply and refill, if necessary.
• Check tubing for kinks and connections for leaks. Notify doctor if you detect any.
• Following the manufacturer's instructions, check balloon for leaks. If you find any, the doctor will replace the balloon.
Possible cause
• Arterial pressure may be damped
Solution
• Check arterial pressure tubing and connections for air bubbles, kinks, or leaks. Flush, if necessary.
Possible cause
• Patient is hypovolemic
Solution
• Notify doctor. Treat hypovolemia, as ordered.

TREATMENT

Continued

Troubleshooting Intraaortic Balloon Pump (IABP) Therapy
Continued

AUGMENTATION CURVE IS ABSENT OR TOO SMALL
Continued

Possible cause
• Patient's cardiac stroke volume exceeds balloon volume
Solution
• Notify doctor. He'll probably begin weaning the patient from the balloon pump.
Possible cause
• Balloon positioned too low in aorta or in a false channel of the aorta
Solution
• Notify doctor. He may remove or reposition the balloon.

AUGMENTATION CURVE IS TOO LARGE

Possible cause
• Too much gas entering balloon
• Balloon too large for patient
Solution
• Decrease gas flow.
• Notify doctor. He may replace balloon with a smaller one.

BALLOON IS DEFLATING PREMATURELY

Possible cause
• Patient has frequent premature ventricular contractions (PVCs)
Solution
• Treat dysrhythmias.

BALLOON LOSES GAS PRESSURE MORE QUICKLY THAN THE ANTICIPATED GRADUAL LOSS

Possible cause
• Balloon leak
Solution
• Stop pumping to investigate.
• Check connections. Following manufacturer's guidelines, check balloon for leaks. Notify the doctor if you find any.

BALLOON INFLATION ALARM SOUNDS

Possible cause
• Depleted gas supply

Continued

TREATMENT

Troubleshooting Intraaortic Balloon Pump (IABP) Therapy
Continued

BALLOON INFLATION
ALARM SOUNDS
Continued

Solution
• Reload the gas system, if necessary.
• Increase the balloon inflation pressure so that it reaches at least +50 mm Hg.

HIGH-VOLUME ALARM
SOUNDS

Possible cause
• Balloon pump volume meter setting exceeds the capacity of balloon
Solution
• Check the volume meter setting. Decrease the setting, if necessary, so it matches the balloon volume.
Possible cause
Balloon catheter improperly connected to console
Solution
• Reconnect the balloon catheter to the console.

ARTERIAL PRESSURE IS
ABSENT OR TOO LOW

Possible cause
• Disconnected balloon catheter or pressure transducer
Solution
• Check and secure all connections.

ARTERIAL PRESSURE IS
TOO HIGH, EXCEEDING
200 mm Hg

Possible cause
• Improperly calibrated pressure transducer
Solution
• Recalibrate the transducer.

ARTERIAL PRESSURE
WAVEFORM IS DAMPED

Possible cause
• Blocked arterial pressure catheter
Solution
• Flush the arterial pressure catheter.

Continued

TREATMENT

Troubleshooting Intraaortic Balloon Pump (IABP) Therapy
Continued

ARTERIAL PRESSURE
WAVEFORM IS OBSCURED
BY INTERFERENCE

Possible cause
• Patient movement

• Jostled catheter
Solution
• Quiet the patient.
• Eliminate any disturbances.

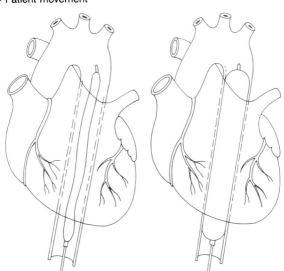

A boost for the ailing heart

Performing Percutaneous Transluminal Coronary Angioplasty (PTCA): Some Indications

The doctor may perform PTCA when your patient has:
• an accesible lesion (noncalcific, concentric, proximal, discrete, preferably in only one vessel) and a history of angina of less than 1 year
• stenosis of a vein graft after coronary artery bypass surgery
• multivessel disease (performed only in selected patients).

He won't perform PTCA if your patient has:
• left main coronary artery lesions
• tortuous, angulated vessels
• multiple or heavily calcified lesions
• poor ventricular function.

PTCA: Weighing Both Sides

PTCA is designed to reduce anginal pain and improve exercise tolerance. But before recommending the procedure, the doctor weighs its disadvantages against its intended benefits. Other factors he evaluates include the following:

Advantages
• Dilates artery immediately
• Requires only about 2 hours to perform (in a catheterization laboratory)
• Requires a shorter hospital stay than coronary artery bypass surgery
• Allows patient to resume activities of daily living almost immediately
• Provides symptomatic relief of angina in patients for whom coronary artery bypass grafting is contraindicated because of advanced age or such preexisting conditions as diabetes, cancer, or previous myocardial infarction.

Disadvantages
• May lead to complications, including AMI, dysrhythmias, coronary vasospasm, or coronary artery dissection with perforation
• Doesn't eliminate the possibility of restenosis
• Necessitates patient preparation for coronary bypass surgery in the event of complications or procedure failure
• Demands patient selectivity on the basis of coronary condition (only one in ten candidates for coronary artery bypass grafting is also a PTCA candidate).

TREATMENT

Coronary Artery Bypass Grafting (CABG)

What's CABG? In this surgical procedure, the doctor grafts a segment of one of the patient's veins (usually a saphenous vein) above and below the coronary artery blockage, providing a bypass that restores blood flow to the myocardium.

If successful, CABG surgery relieves pain and improves myocardial performance.

Indications and Contraindications

TREATMENT

If CABG is successful, it improves blood supply to the heart and relieves anginal pain, improving the patient's exercise tolerance and quality of life. But, like any major surgical procedure, CABG has risks and disadvantages. It requires a 10- to 14-day hospital stay with scrupulous postoperative care. Complications can develop. The benefits of surgery may be only temporary. And postpericardiotomy syndrome (increased chest pain, fatigue, sinus tachycardia, or palpitations) develops in up to 30% of patients.

The doctor will consider these indications and contraindications before arriving at one of the following decisions.

He will probably perform CABG surgery for a patient with:
• atherosclerosis affecting one or more coronary arteries (if the patient's experiencing severe angina despite medical therapy).
• an AMI that develops during cardiac catheterization, arteriography, or PTCA.
• an AMI with a papillary muscle rupture, septal rupture, or persistent pain.
• some uncontrollable ventricular dysrhythmias, particularly when a left ventricular aneurysm is present.
• left main coronary artery stenosis greater than 50%, narrowing of several coronary arteries, or triple-vessel coronary artery disease.

The doctor won't perform CABG surgery for a patient with:
• an uncomplicated transmural infarct.
• severe left ventricular dysfunction.
• distal coronary arteries that are diseased and too small for successful graft placement.

Patients for Pacing

In the early days of pacemaking, the sole indication was complete atrioventricular block leading to Stokes-Adams attacks. Nowadays, doctors implant pacemakers for many conduction defects, ranging from complete to partial and/or intermittent AV block. Accepted indications include:

• complete AV block lasting 1 to 3 weeks or more following acute myocardial infarction
• complete AV block associated with congestive heart failure or cerebral or renal insufficiency that improves with temporary pacing
• persistent AV block following cardiac surgery
• need for prophylaxis following cardiac surgery
• incomplete AV block (Mobitz Type II or advanced second-degree block)
• symptomatic bilateral bundle branch block
• symptomatic sinus bradycardia, with or without AV block
• sinus arrest or sinoatrial block
• sick sinus syndrome
• trifascicular block
• atrial tachycardia
• need for improved cardiac output.

Pacemaker Tips

• Explain to the patient why the procedure is necessary and how it will be performed.
• Show the patient a pacemaker; explain how it works.
• Watch him carefully after insertion to verify that the pacemaker is functioning properly and effectively.
• Watch for loss of capture, competition, signs of perforation, thrombophlebitis, or skin infection.
• Tell the patient and his family at what rate his pacemaker is set.

PACEMAKERS

Pacemaker Parts

A pacemaker has two basic components:

• *a pulse generator* containing a power source and electronic circuitry. A temporary pacemaker's pulse generator is external; because the pacemaker is intended for short-term use only, it's powered by a standard alkaline or mercury battery.

Most permanent pacemakers are powered by lithium batteries, which last 7 to 10 years. Nuclear batteries are also available.

• *one or two pacing leads*, consisting of a wire catheter with one or two electrodes on the catheter tip. Leads are made in various shapes to aid positioning; a *J* shape is one common type. Depending on the number of leads and their positions, the pacemaker can pace the atria, the ventricles, or both.

A pacing lead can be surgically implanted on the heart's epicardial surface—typically after open heart surgery. Or it can be threaded through a vein to the heart's endocardial surface, where it lodges. Some leads screw into the endocardial surface to help maintain proper placement.

Learning About Pacing Electrodes

The pacing electrode is the part of the pacemaker system that runs from the pacer into the heart. It transmits the patient's cardiac rhythm to the pacer. The pacer then delivers a stimulus to the heart via this same electrode. Two main types of electrodes are now in use: unipolar and bipolar.

Electrical current can flow only when there's a positive and negative pole. The *unipolar* electrode gets its name from the single pole imbedded in its tip. The other pole that's necessary for electrical conduction is built into the casing of the implanted pacer. The unipolar electrode produces tall EKG pacing spikes because of the distance between the two poles.

The *bipolar* electrode has both poles imbedded in the electrode itself. The bipolar electrode produces short EKG pacing spikes because the two poles are close together.

Many styles of electrode tips are available. Which one the doctor selects depends on the mode of pacing and the insertion site.

Types of Pacemakers

Temporary
Temporary pacemakers are inserted via the subclavian, jugular, antecubital, or femoral vein. Under fluoroscopic guidance, the doctor threads the catheter through a vein to the right ventricle.

Permanent
Permanent pacemakers are inserted transvenously via the cephalic or subclavian vein into the right atrium or the apex of the right ventricle. The newest pacemaker modes allow for both atrial and ventricular pacing. The internal pulse generator is usually implanted in a pocket the doctor forms in the anterior chest.

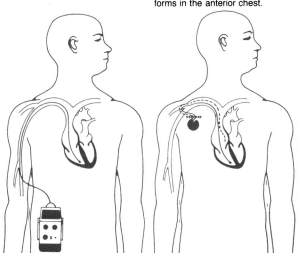

Types of Pacemakers

A three-letter identification code for implantable cardiac pacemakers helps you to sort out their complex characteristics. The first letter identifies the paced chamber: V stands for ventricle, A for atrium, and D for double (atrium and ventricle). The second letter identifies the sensed chamber: A or V. The third letter identifies the response mode: I for inhibited and T for triggered. The letter O means no specific comment is applicable.

Pacemakers are commonly grouped by pacing mode:

• **Fixed-rate pacemakers** (AOO, VOO, DOO) keep a steady rate (usually 70 beats/minute) regardless of the patient's own cardiac impulses. Because such pacing interferes with normal cardiac activity, it may become dangerous when threshold for ventricular fibrillation is low (for example, after MI). Fixed-rate pacemakers are rarely used.

• **QRS-inhibited pacemaker** (VVI), a demand pacemaker with an inhibited response mode, prevents firing of an impulse when the pacemaker senses an R wave.

• **QRS-triggered pacemaker** (VVT) fires in the absolute refractory period when it senses the R wave. So, when natural cardiac rhythm is adequate, this pacemaker fires but causes no cardiac response. But, if cardiac rate falls below the pacemaker's preset rate, the artificial discharge stimulates the myocardium.

• **Atrial synchronized pacemaker** (VAT) uses an atrial electrode to sense normal atrial depolarization. After an appropriate delay to permit atrial transport, it triggers a ventricular electrode to pace the ventricle. If the atrial rate exceeds 130 beats/minute, the pacemaker transmits every other impulse to the ventricle. If the rate falls below 60, it initiates fixed pacing at 60 beats/minute.

• **Atrioventricular sequential pacing** (DVI) imitates the normal sequence of electrical activity in the heart, maintaining cardiac output 22% higher than conventional pacemakers. It uses two separate

Continued

PACEMAKERS

Types of Pacemakers
Continued

electrodes to pace the atrium and ventricle in sequence. However, it's inhibited by ventricular activity.

Pacemakers can also be grouped according to their use:
• **Atrial pacemakers** are used when AV conduction is intact, especially for symptomatic bradycardia and sick sinus syndrome, with or without CHF and low cardiac output. Rapid atrial pacing is helpful to end intractable supraventricular and ventricular tachydysrhythmias. Atrial pacemakers are hemodynamically superior to ventricular pacemakers because they maintain ventricular filling. But, maintaining electrode contact with atrial tissue isn't easy. Reliable lead fixation can cure this problem.
• **Atrial synchronous** are commonly used when complete heart block prevents use of an atrial pacemaker or when another condition prevents ventricular pacing because the patient needs atrial contraction to maintain cardiac output.
• **Ventricular pacemakers** are primarily (95%) used to treat sinus bradycardia.

Setting the Stimulation Threshold

The stimulation threshold must be determined to maintain myocardial contractions. As ordered
• Set the pacemaker's sensitivity control to *fixed* or *demand*. Run EKG monitor strips and note the milliamperes (MA) on each strip as you adjust the MA level.
• Increase the rate above the patient's heart rate.
• Increase the MA, and watch the EKG for "capture". Stop increasing the MA when 100% capture is achieved. Slowly decrease the MA until you lose capture.
• Record the threshold as *the lowest MA that achieves capture.*
• Set the MA and rate.

DDD Versus VVI: Comparing Two Types

The newest pacemaker type—known by its Inter-Society Commission for Heart Disease code, DDD—paces the atria and ventricles and senses in both chambers, mimicking normal cardiac function. Also called a *universal* pacemaker, a DDD pacemaker stimulates an atrial contraction if the sinoatrial node fails to do so. Then, if the ventricles don't respond spontaneously, it stimulates a ventricular contraction. This system ensures atrial contribution to ventricular filling; it also provides a backup in case the ventricles fail to respond properly.

Because it mimics normal cardiac electrical function, the DDD has these benefits:
• increases ventricular filling time, which in turn increases stroke volume
• increases force of myocardial contractions
• minimizes regurgitation by allowing complete atrioventricular (AV) valve closure.

Although the DDD pacing system has compelling advantages, it's not indicated for everyone. You're more apt to encounter the VVI (ventricular demand) pacemaker, which senses and paces the ventricle at a set rate unless inhibited by a spontaneous QRS complex. By doing so, it prevents heart rate from slowing dangerously but permits the heart to pace itself when the spontaneous rate is higher than the preset pacemaker rate.

To help you recall what the DDD pacing system does and when, remember that the DDD pacemaker gives patients what they require when they require it. For more detailed information, be sure to read the manufacturer's manual.

The VVI pacing system, although helpful for patients with third-degree AV block, has several disadvantages:
• Because pacemaker activity doesn't mimic natural function, it doesn't vary with exercise or rest. Also, paced beats are ectopic, so they don't travel along the normal conduction pathway. This can reduce cardiac output significantly.
• Lack of atrioventricular synchrony may contribute to reduced cardiac output and pacemaker syndrome. In addition, spontaneous atrial contractions that occur simultaneously with paced ventricular contractions may cause mitral and tricuspid regurgitation, producing dyspnea.

Assessing Capture

When the pacemaker sends an electrical impulse to the heart, it appears on the EKG strip as a vertical line, commonly called the pacemaker spike. When the spike is followed by a QRS complex or P wave, *capture* has occurred.

If the pacemaker electrode rests in the ventricle, you'll see a spike in front of every QRS complex that's stimulated by the pacemaker. These complexes appear wide and bizarre—similar to those caused by premature ventricular contractions, except that they won't be early. If the electrode's

in the atrium, a spike before a P wave indicates that capture has occurred; the P wave may be inverted or may differ in shape from a spontaneous P wave. If electrodes are pacing both the atria and ventricles, you'll see spikes before both QRS complexes and P waves.

Because spikes may not appear in every EKG lead, verify capture by checking more than one lead. A lead that reveals pacing spikes well is aVR, because the QRS complexes are small and less likely to obscure the spike.

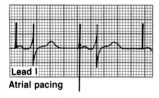

Lead I
Atrial pacing

Pacemaker spike

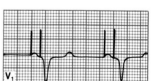

V₁
Atrial and ventricular pacing

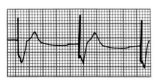

Ventricular pacing

PACEMAKERS

Guide to Pacemaker Mode and Placement

Years ago, differentiating pacemaker modes was easy. The pacemaker was set to fire into a patient's ventricle either at a fixed rate or at a demand rate. But today, pacemaker modes and placement are not so simple. Of course, you may still employ fixed or demand pacemakers. But you'll probably use a variation or combination of these basic modes, such as a pacemaker that senses one chamber but fires at a fixed rate into another (Demand example B). Or you may use a new mode entirely, such as a physiological pacemaker that fires into the atrium and ventricle, as needed, to synchronize right-sided heart contractions.

PACEMAKER MODE	DESCRIPTION	ELECTRODE PLACEMENT
FIXED (example A)	Pacemaker delivers an electrical impulse at a predetermined rate to the atrium or the ventricle (depending on electrode placement). Pacemaker rate remains fixed regardless of the patient's intrinsic heart rate.	Right ventricle or, in rare cases, right atrium
DEMAND (example A)	Pacemaker senses patient's ventricular contractions (represented by the QRS complex) and only delivers an electrical stimulus (at a predetermined rate) if no contraction occurs.	Right ventricle

PACEMAKERS

Several ways exist to differentiate pacemakers. Each manufacturer assigns its own designations to its pacemakers. Your hospital may use those designations. Or your hospital may identify pacemaker types and operating modes by using a letter code. Codes vary from hospital to hospital, so if your hospital employs one, make sure you learn it.

This chart features basic pacemaker modes and a few variations. To learn about your patient's pacemaker, consult the manufacturer's booklet.

ADVANTAGES	DISADVANTAGES	EFFECT ON EKG WAVEFORM (S INDICATES PACEMAKER SPIKE)
• Simple circuitry and mechanism	• Does not accommodate changes in patient's intrinsic heart rate • May cause cardiac dysrhythmias • Atrium electrode placement will work only if the patient has an intact electrical conduction system	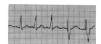
• Accommodates changes in patient's intrinsic heart rate • Usually does not cause cardiac dysrhythmias • Battery often lasts longer than with fixed mode	• Complicated circuitry and mechanism	

PACEMAKERS

Continued

Guide to Pacemaker Mode and Placement
Continued

PACEMAKER MODE	DESCRIPTION	ELECTRODE PLACEMENT
FIXED (example B)	Pacemaker senses the patient's ventricular contractions (the QRS complex) and fires continuously. If heart rate falls below a predetermined rate, this firing replaces the QRS complex. If the heart rate stays at or goes faster than a predetermined rate, the pacemaker keeps pace with the contractions, firing harmlessly into the patient's intrinsic QRS complex.	Right ventricle
DEMAND (example B)	Pacemaker senses atrial contractions, waits a predetermined interval, then fires into the ventricle. If no atrial contraction is present, the pacemaker fires into the atrium and the ventricle.	Right atrium and right ventricle.

PACEMAKERS

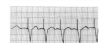

ADVANTAGES	DISADVANTAGES	EFFECT ON EKG WAVEFORM (S INDICATES PACE-MAKER SPIKE)
• Accommodates changes in patient's intrinsic heart rate • Usually does not cause cardiac dysrhythmias	• Complicated circuitry and mechanism	
• Accommodates changes in patient's intrinsic heart rate • Usually does not cause cardiac dysrhythmias	• Complicated circuitry and mechanism	

PACEMAKERS

Assisting with Temporary Pacemaker Insertion

Suppose a patient comes into the ED with acute dysrhythmias from a myocardial infarction. First you may administer antiarrhythmic drugs, as ordered. But if the drugs don't work, the doctor may insert a temporary pacemaker. It electrically stimulates the heart muscle to maintain adequate cardiac rate and rhythm. Here's how a pacemaker works and what you need to know to assist with its insertion:

Pacemaker mechanics

Temporary pacemakers may be inserted for either atrial or ventricular pacing (more common in an emergency).

To insert a pacemaker, the doctor threads a pacing catheter through the patient's subclavian, femoral, jugular, or antecubital vein. Once the catheter's in place, resting at the apex of the right heart, he connects it to an external pacemaker that's set on either a fixed or a demand mode. The patient's stimulation threshold determines the pacemaker's milliamp setting.

Doctors select demand mode more often than fixed mode. This is because fixed mode interferes with a patient's intrinsic heart rate and may cause ventricular tachycardia or ventricular fibrillation.

Equipment
- Skin-preparation supplies
- Sterile gloves, towels
- 5-ml syringe and needle
- Introducer wire
- Sterile suture tray
- Antiseptic ointment, sterile gauze dressing, nonallergenic tape
- Temporary pacer and pacing catheter

Nursing considerations
- Make sure a signed consent form has been obtained before the procedure.
- Gather the necessary equipment and assist the doctor with inserting and setting the pacemaker.
- Watch the EKG monitor for premature ventricular contractions, ventricular tachycardia, or ventricular fibrillation caused by electrode irritation of the ventricle. Have lidocaine and a defibrillator ready.
- Record the pacemaker's mode, rate, and stimulation threshold on your patient's chart and nursing-care plan.
- Make sure the pacing spike is in the correct position on the EKG waveform—just before the QRS complex (see illustration).
- Continuously monitor the patient's EKG. Notify the doctor if you see ventricular ectopic beats.

Continued

Assisting with Temporary Pacemaker Insertion
Continued

• Check the patient's vital signs and level of consciousness hourly.
• Auscultate the patient's lungs and heart for rales, decreased breath sounds, or friction rubs every 2 to 4 hours.
• If you move the patient, elevate the affected limb to immobilize it and to ensure adequate circulation. Use a drawsheet to reposition the patient in bed.
• Change the dressings using sterile technique, and apply antibiotic ointment.
• Check the insertion site for signs of infection and for bleeding.

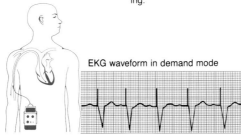

EKG waveform in demand mode

Special Consideration

Special considerations: Watch for signs of pacemaker malfunction. Make sure all electrical equipment is grounded with three-pronged plugs inserted in the right receptacles. Also, cover all exposed metal parts of the pacemaker setup with nonconductive tape, or place the pacing unit in a dry rubber surgical glove. Instruct the patient not to use an electric razor or any other nonessential electrical equipment. If emergency defibrillation should be necessary, make sure the pacemaker can withstand this procedure before starting it; if not, disconnect it. Protect the pacemaker and its connections from moisture. If the patient is disoriented or uncooperative, restrain his arms to prevent accidental removal of pacemaker wires. If any evidence of infection is present during catheter implantation, culture disposable pacemaker catheter tips after they're removed.

Interpreting a Pacemaker Code

As this diagram illustrates, the DVI pacemaker paces both the atrium and ventricle, senses only ventricular activity, and is inhibited by intrinsic ventricular impulses.

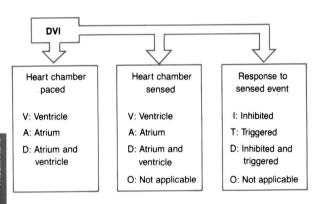

Heart chamber paced	Heart chamber sensed	Response to sensed event
V: Ventricle	V: Ventricle	I: Inhibited
A: Atrium	A: Atrium	T: Triggered
D: Atrium and ventricle	D: Atrium and ventricle	D: Inhibited and triggered
	O: Not applicable	O: Not applicable

Caring for Pacemaker Patients

If your patient has a temporary or permanent pacemaker, you'll need to provide special nursing care and comprehensive patient teaching.

Temporary pacemaker care

If a patient has a temporary pacemaker, record on his chart the date and method of insertion, the location (atrial or ventricular) of the pacemaker, and its type, rate, threshold (MA) settings, times turned on or off, and frequency of use.

To maintain pacemaker function, continuously monitor the EKG for frequency of pacing need, maintenance of preset rate, capture, sensing, and paced QRS or P configuration. After insertion of a temporary pacemaker and every 8 hours thereafter, check the connections, battery, pulse at the insertion site, and consistency between the pacemaker setting and the actual rate and stimulation and sensitivity thresholds when the pacemaker is on and off. Every 24 hours or as indicated, check the threshold; every 4 hours or as indicated, check vital signs and the sense/pace needle.

To maintain equipment, place a plastic cover over the dials to keep the box and wires dry. Clean the box with water or alcohol, or gas-sterilize it, but never autoclave it. Clean nondisposable catheters in bactericidal solution, and then gas-sterilize them. Before defibrillation, find out if the doctor wants the pacemaker disconnected.

To prevent infection at the insertion site, cleanse the skin with antiseptic solution and apply antibiotic ointment and dry, sterile dressings daily. To prevent ulceration of underlying tissue, pad the area beneath the wires. Inspect the site every 4 hours for tenderness, redness, swelling, and discoloration. When you remove the catheter, culture the tip if it has been in place for over 1 week, if signs of infection are present, or if insertion was traumatic.

To prevent microshock, insulate the external metallic parts of the pacing catheter. When you handle these parts, wear dry rubber or plastic gloves. Protect these parts of newer models by imbedding them in the insulated pacemaker terminals or by covering them with clear tape or a dry,
Continued

PACEMAKERS

Caring for Pacemaker Patients
Continued

surgical rubber glove. Make sure all equipment is properly grounded, using a three-prong plug; don't use adapters. Don't use extension cords or equipment that has frayed wires or other signs of disrepair. If you're not sure equipment is in good condition, check with the hospital electrician. Prevent the patient from contacting metal. Warn him not to touch a television set. Don't touch the patient or his bed while touching electrical equipment. Avoid using electrical beds that are not specifically approved; unplug lamps attached to metal beds; and make sure electrical equipment, such as a respirator, doesn't touch the bed. Place a "microshock precaution" sign over the bed, and explain the sign to the patient and his family.

To maintain the patient's comfort, give medication for pain, as ordered. If the patient has pain or discomfort in his legs or arms, check pulse and perfusion distal to the cutdown every 8 hours. Position the affected extremity comfortably, and to avoid stiffness, help the patient gently exercise it regularly.

Permanent pacemaker care
If a patient has a permanent pacemaker, record on his chart the date and location of the insertion, the manufacturer's model and serial numbers for the generator and leads, the set rate, EKG tracings with and without a magnet held over the generator, amplitude of pacemaker artifact, and threshold measurements at insertion.

To maintain pacemaker function, continuously monitor the patient's EKG for the first 24 hours; then analyze the EKG every 4 hours for maintenance of the preset rate, capture, paced QRS configuration, amplitude of pacemaker artifact, sensing, competition, and ventricular dysrhythmias. Check consistency against baseline values.

Every 4 hours, check blood pressure, respiration, and temperature; count apical and radial pulses for 1 minute. Every 2 hours, quickly check these pulses. Report any rates below the pacing rate or an apical-radial pulse deficit.

Watch for signs of pacemaker failure (decreased blood pressure, decreased urinary output, Stokes-Adams syndrome, palpitations, chest pains, dyspnea and fatigue, lightheadedness). Also, watch for signs of pacing catheter displacement (intermittent or complete pacing failure, abnormal pacemaker stimulation).

Continued

Caring for Pacemaker Patients
Continued

To avoid such displacement, make sure the patient doesn't raise his arms above the shoulder until the doctor orders range-of-motion (ROM) exercises, usually around the third postoperative day. Enforce bed rest for 24 hours and reduced activity for another 48 hours.

To make sure that equipment (batteries, pacing catheter) is working well, watch for ventricular premature beats, frequency, and coupling interval; and check for sensing or competition.

To avoid infection, inspect the insertion site at regular intervals and whenever the patient reports discomfort. Check for signs of infection, skin breakdown, or hematoma. Check temperature every 4 hours. If a closed-wound drain is in use, empty it every 8 hours or as needed. When you remove the pressure dressing, replace it with a sterile dressing. Change the sterile dressing daily. Give antibiotics for 5 to 7 days after implantation, as ordered.

To promote comfort, assist and encourage the patient to begin ROM exercises for the affected shoulder, as ordered, usually 5 to 7 days after pacemaker insertion. Administer an analgesic, as needed.

Questions Pacemaker Patients May Ask

- What am I allowed to do now that I have a pacemaker?
- Can I return to work?
- What daily medical care must I practice?
- Do I have to check my pulse often?
- Can water hurt my pacemaker?
- How do I care for my incision?
- What else should I watch for?
- Can I travel?
- May I fly in a plane?
- Can electrical equipment harm me?
- How long will my pacemaker last?
- What happens if it stops working?

PACEMAKERS

Teaching Your Patient About His Pacemaker

You confront two challenges when you teach your patient about his cardiac pacemaker. The first is to gear the sessions to your patient's intellectual capacity and interest level. The second is to recognize and allay his fears. These fears can range from an obvious one of death if the pacemaker fails to a subtle one of altered body image.

Begin your first session by reviewing the facts contained in the heart and pacemaker booklets that you gave your patient before the insertion. As before, you may want to show him a heart model, pacer, and electrode to demonstrate what you're explaining.

Your patient's ID card
While he's in the hospital, your patient will probably be issued a temporary ID card stating that he has a pacemaker. Explain that he must carry the card with him at all times. He'll be sent a permanent ID card after he returns home. Also, provide him with the information he needs to order an ID bracelet. Encourage him to buy one and wear it at all times.

Does your patient have a nuclear pacemaker? If he plans to travel abroad, he must inform the pacemaker manufacturer of his travel itinerary, means of travel, and the name of the doctor supervising his care. This is a requirement of the Nuclear Regulatory Commission.

Tell your patient that airport security systems will detect his pacemaker. To board the plane, he may have to show airline officials his ID card.

Teach your patient to take his pulse
After he's discharged from the hospital, your patient should take his pulse daily, preferably when he's sitting in a comfortable chair, or sitting up in bed. Make sure he obtains a *resting* pulse rate; for example, just before getting out of bed each morning. He should take his pulse for at least 1 minute.

For your patient to assess his pulse rate, he must understand his pacemaker mode. If the patient has a demand pacemaker, his intrinsic heart rate may be higher than the set rate of the pacemaker. This may cause him undue concern. Remind him that his pacemaker is an emergency backup system—for example, if his heart rate should decrease while he's asleep, the pacemaker will take over and maintain his heart rate at the predetermined level. Inform him of what pulse discrepancy is acceptable, what is not, and who to call when the discrepancy is unacceptable. Give him written instructions.

PACEMAKERS

Asking the Right Questions

If you suspect that your patient's pacemaker is malfunctioning, assess the situation by answering the following questions.

• What's the patient's condition? As always, your first step is to determine whether he's in distress and needs emergency intervention. Assess for hypotension and other signs of low cardiac output.

• Why was his pacemaker inserted, and what's it supposed to do? The patient's history will tell you about his underlying condition. If possible, refer to the patient's pacemaker card for details on the pacemaker's capabilities. Or use the pacemaker's programmer to identify the pacemaker's settings.

Note: If no programmer is available, obtain a chest X-ray. It may enable you to read the pacemaker's model and serial number.

• What is the pacemaker doing now? Obtain an EKG and assess pacing, capture, and sensing.

• Is the malfunction contributing to the patient's symptoms?

• Can it be adjusted? If it's a demand pacemaker, it can be adjusted with a programmer.

• Does it need adjusting now? Refer to guidelines set by the doctor; notify him if appropriate.

• Should part or all of the pacemaker equipment be replaced? If so, prepare the patient for surgery.

A Glossary of Terms

Capture. A pacemaker's ability to cause atrial and/or ventricular depolarization.

Competition. Paced beats occurring simultaneously with spontaneous beats—a risk with fixed-rate pacemakers.

Noncapture. Failure of a pacemaker to cause atrial and/or ventricular depolarization

Oversensing. Inappropriate pacemaker inhibition from the pacemaker's sensing and being inhibited by something other than intrinisic atrial and/or ventricular depolarization.

Pacemaker syndrome. Fatigue, dizziness, and dyspnea associated with a fall in sinus rate at the onset of ventricular pacing. Caused by loss of AV synchrony, it may follow exercise.

Sensing. A pacemaker's ability to detect atrial and/or ventricular depolarization.

Threshold (stimulation threshold). The electrical energy needed to obtain capture.

Dealing with Cardiac Complications Related to Pacemakers

PATIENT PROBLEM	CAUSE	SOLUTION
Premature ventricular contractions, ventricular tachycardia, ventricular fibrillation	• Myocardium irritated during implant	• Doctor will order medication, such as lidocaine hydrochloride (Xylocaine*), to treat irritability.
Myocardial hemorrhage	• Electrode tip placed in the epicardium	• If cardiac tamponade has occurred, the doctor may perform an emergency pericardiocentesis.
Swelling, redness, drainage, and pain at insertion site	• Local or systemic infection	• Doctor will probably order antibiotics. May remove lead wire and insert it at new site.
Fluid accumulation, pacer migration, and/or pocket erosion (for permanent pacemaker only)	• Body rejection	• Doctor will withdraw fluid with a needle and syringe. May reposition pacer.
Muscle twitching at the pocket site (for permanent pacemakers only)	• Misplaced electrode tip	• Doctor will pull back slightly on lead wire to reposition electrode tip.
Rapid hiccuping	• Misplaced electrode tip stimulating diaphragm	• Doctor will pull back slightly on lead wire to reposition electrode tip.

*Available in United States and in Canada

Testing and Reprogramming

Your patient has a ventricular demand (VVI) pacemaker set at a rate of 70 beats/minute. The past few hours, he's begun to experience the same symptoms that prompted pacemaker insertion: chest pain, dizziness, palpitations, and fatigue. Your initial assessment findings lead you to suspect pacemaker malfunction. But how can you be sure?

Testing. First, obtain a 12-lead EKG tracing and a chest X-ray, if ordered. Depending on your findings, the doctor may then want you to perform a magnet test to assess whether the pacemaker is firing properly. If so, take the following steps.

Caution: Never attempt a magnet test unless your patient is connected to a cardiac monitor or EKG machine and you have a defibrillator and other emergency equipment nearby. Although complications are rare, the test may trigger ventricular fibrillation.

• Hold the magnet 1″ (2.5 cm) from the implanted pulse generator. A magnetically controlled reed switch in the pulse generator will close, causing the pacemaker to revert to fixed-rate firing.

Note: Avoid moving the magnet excessively, or you may damage the reed switch.

• After 1 minute, withdraw the magnet. The reed switch will open, allowing demand pacing to resume.

• Calculate the pacing rate by counting the pacemaker spikes on an EKG strip. If you count 70 for a 1-minute period, the pacemaker is firing properly.

Note: Don't expect a QRS complex to follow every spike; if the spike falls on a refractory period, a QRS complex won't appear.

Reprogramming. To change various operational settings, including pacing rate, stimulus output, pulse duration or amplitude, sensitivity, PR interval (refractory period), and pacing mode, the doctor (or a specially trained nurse or technician) will use an external programmer supplied by the pacemaker's manufacturer. *Continued*

PACEMAKERS

Testing and Reprogramming
Continued

To compare the pacemaker's programmed settings with actual function, the doctor simply presses buttons on the programmer; the information appears on a display panel. With this equipment, he can find out if the pacemaker's circuitry, battery, and electrode are working properly.

Some programmers use telemetry to identify the pacemaker's programmer settings and evaluate how it's functioning.

Pacemaker Function: Phone Check

Reassure your patient that checking pacemaker function is as easy as picking up the phone. For example, the Medtronic pacemaker uses a Medtronic Model 9408 Tele-Trace Transmitter to telephone an EKG signal to the doctor's office or clinic.

Explain to your patient that at an appointed time he'll call a predetermined phone number. Then, he'll rest a small rectangular transmitter against his bare chest and put the telephone's mouth-piece against the transmitter's speaker. The transmitter will detect electrical signals generated by the patient's pacemaker and convert them to sound waves. The telephone receiver will then send these sound waves to a receiver in the office or clinic, which will convert them to an EKG readout strip. By examining the strip, the doctor will be able to evaluate pacemaker function.

Troubleshooting Pacemaker Problems

NONCAPTURE

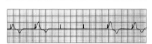

Lead I

Signs and symptoms
• Bradycardia
• Hypotension, dyspnea, chest pain, dizziness, fatigue, and other signs of low cardiac output
• On an EKG, pacemaker spikes aren't followed by QRS complexes (if the electrode is ventricular) or by P waves (if the electrode is atrial).

Possible Causes
• Electrode tip out of position
• Pacemaker voltage too low
• Lead wire fracture
• Battery depletion
• Edema or scar tissue formation at electrode tip
• Myocardial perforation by lead wire

Intervention
• Reposition the patient on his side; if the electrode tip is malpositioned, this may correct the problem.
• Reprogram the pacemaker to increase voltage (MAs), if necessary.
• Obtain a chest X-ray to check for electrode wire fracture, malpositioned electrode tip, or myocardial perforation.
• If the patient's heart rate is extremely slow, administer a positive chronotropic drug (such as isoproterenol hydrochloride [Isuprel*]) or atropine sulfate), as ordered.
• Prepare the patient for surgery to replace or reposition equipment, if necessary.
• Monitor the patient for signs and symptoms of cardiac tamponade (such as hypotension, tachycardia, and pulsus paradoxus), a possible result of myocardial perforation.

Continued

PACEMAKERS

Unmarked trade names available in the United States only
*Also available in Canada

Troubleshooting Pacemaker Problems
Continued

PACEMAKER RATE TOO SLOW OR PACEMAKER STOPS PACING

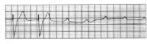

V₁

Signs and symptoms
• Bradycardia or a heart rate that's slower than the preset pacemaker rate
• Hypotension and other signs of low cardiac output
Possible causes
• Battery failure
• Circuitry failure
Intervention
• Replace the battery or temporary pacemaker generator (for a temporary pacemaker).
• Prepare the patient for surgery to replace equipment (for a permanent pacemaker).

NONSENSING

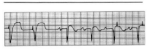

V₁

Signs and symptoms
• Palpitations, skipped beats, ventricular tachycardia, or ventricular fibrillation (rare)
• On an EKG, spikes may fall on T waves, or they may fall regularly but at points where they shouldn't appear.
Possible causes
• Battery depletion
• Electrode tip out of position
• Lead wire fracture
• Increased sensing threshold from edema or fibrosis at electrode tip
Intervention
• Reposition the patient on his side; this may reposition the electrode tip.
• Obtain a chest X-ray to check for lead wire fracture or electrode malposition.
• Replace the battery, if necessary.
• Prepare the patient for surgery to replace or reposition the lead wire, if necessary.
• Adjust the pacemaker's sensitivity setting, if necessary.

Continued

PACEMAKERS

Troubleshooting Pacemaker Problems
Continued

OVERSENSING

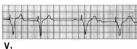

V_1

Signs and symptoms
• Pacemaker pacing at a rate slower than the set rate
• No paced beats at all (even though spontaneous rate is slower than the pacemaker's set rate)

Possible causes
• Myopotentials (with unipolar leads only). The pacemaker may sense (and be inhibited by) skeletal muscle contractions.
• Electromagnetic interference

Intervention
• Perform the external magnet test, as ordered.
• Prepare the patient for surgical insertion of a bipolar lead, if ordered.
• Adjust the pacemaker's sensitivity setting, if necessary.

PREMATURE VENTRICULAR CONTRACTIONS (PVCs)

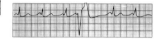

Lead II

Signs and symptoms
• Patient complaining of skipped beats
• PVCs visible on an EKG

Possible cause
• Electrode causing irritable ventricular focus
Note: PVCs occur normally within the first 24 hours after pacemaker insertion; they're not treated during this time unless they cause symptoms.

Intervention
• Initiate continuous cardiac monitoring.
• Administer antiarrhythmic drugs, as ordered.
• Prepare the patient for surgery to reposition the lead wire, if necessary.

Continued

Troubleshooting Pacemaker Problems
Continued

PACEMAKER TACHYCARDIA

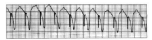

V₃

Signs and symptoms
● On an EKG, tachycardia with pacemaker spikes preceding each QRS complex
Possible cause
● Retrograde conduction through the AV node, repolarizing the atria and triggering rapid pacemaker firing; most common with DDD pacemakers
Intervention
● Slow the heart rate by holding a magnet over the pulse generator; this converts a demand pacemaker into a fixed-rate pacemaker.
Note: You may have to continue holding the magnet in place until the pacemaker is reprogrammed.
● Monitor the patient for ventricular tachycardia and fibrillation.

● The doctor or a specially trained nurse or technician will reprogram the pacemaker's PR interval to increase the refractory period.

DIAPHRAGMATIC STIMULATION

Signs and symptoms
● Hiccups
● Artifact on an EKG
Possible causes
● Stimulation of phrenic nerve by electrode tip
● Myocardial perforation by lead wire
● Excessive pacemaker voltage (MAs)
Intervention
● Reposition patient; his hiccups may disappear when he lies on his side.
● Closely monitor the patient for signs of cardiac tamponade.
● Decrease the MAs, if necessary.
● Prepare the patient for surgery to reposition the lead wire, if necessary.

Keeping Track of Cholesterol

To help control the amount of cholesterol in your blood, the doctor wants you to limit your cholesterol intake to less than 300 mg a day. Make sure you stay within this limit by using the following chart, which shows the approximate cholesterol content of some common foods.

	SERVING SIZE	CHOLESTEROL CONTENT
Breads		
biscuit	1	17 mg
bread slice or roll	any amount	0 mg
French toast	1	130 mg
pancake	1	38 mg
saltine crackers	any amount	0 mg
sweet roll	1	25 mg
Cheeses		
American	1 oz	30 mg
cottage cheese		
creamed	1 cup	45 mg
uncreamed	1 cup	16 mg
mozzarella	1 oz	18 mg
Muenster	1 oz	25 mg
Parmesan	1 oz	25 mg
provolone	1 oz	27 mg
ricotta	1 oz	14 mg
Swiss	1 oz	28 mg
Cooking oils		
lard	1 tbsp	12 mg
margarine	any amount	0 mg
vegetable oils	any amount	0 mg
Desserts		
angel food cake	any amount	0 mg
baked custard	1 cup	275 mg
chocolate cake	1 slice	32 mg
sherbet	any amount	0 mg

REHABILITATION

Continued

Keeping Track of Cholesterol
Continued

	SERVING SIZE	CHOLESTEROL CONTENT
Fish		
clams	1 oz	13 mg
haddock	1 oz	23 mg
herring	1 oz	32 mg
oysters	1 oz	19 mg
salmon	1 oz	18 mg
scallops	1 oz	15 mg
shrimp	1 oz	57 mg
trout	1 oz	21 mg
tuna	1 oz	21 mg
Meat		
bacon	2 slices	15 mg
beef (lean)	1 oz	36 mg
beef (liver)	1 oz	123 mg
lamb	1 oz	37 mg
pork (ham)	1 oz	33 mg
pork (sausages)	1 oz	27 mg
veal	1 oz	38 mg
Milk and dairy products		
butter	1 tbsp	30 mg
egg white	any amount	0 mg
egg yolk	1 egg	245 mg
ice cream	½ cup	25 mg
ice milk	½ cup	5 mg
skim milk	1 cup	5 mg
whole milk	1 cup	32 mg
Poultry		
chicken (light meat with skin)	1 oz	22 mg
turkey (light meat with skin)	1 oz	23 mg

Continued

Keeping Track of Cholesterol
Continued

SERVING SIZE	CHOLESTEROL CONTENT	
Miscellaneous		
chocolate sauce	any amount	0 mg
coconut	any amount	0 mg
gravy	¼ cup	18 mg
low-fat cookies	any amount	0 mg
popcorn (unbuttered)	any amount	0 mg
potatoes	any amount	0 mg
white sauce	¼ cup	29 mg

This teaching aid may be reproduced by office copier for distribution to patients. © 1985, Springhouse Corporation.

Cutting Back on Cholesterol

Help your patient stick to his low-fat diet by giving him the following advice:
• When shopping, read product labels for fat content. Buy only foods made with polyunsaturated or vegetable fats.
• Drink skim milk and use skim milk products.
• Follow your doctor's recommendation for the number of egg yolks you can safely eat weekly.

• Limit your intake of beef, ham, and pork.
• Trim off as much fat from meat as possible before cooking it.
• Don't fry foods.
• If you boil or simmer meat, immediately remove it from the cooking liquid when it's done.
• After preparing soups or gravies, chill them; then skim off the fat.
• Avoid creamy or cheesy sauces.

REHABILITATION

Low-Sodium Diet for the MI Patient

An MI patient must watch his diet. His doctor will most likely restrict his sodium intake, so before he leaves the hospital explain the importance of avoiding the following:
• salted "snack" foods, such as potato chips and peanuts
• canned soups and vegetables
• dried fruits
• delicatessen foods, especially lox and ham
• prepared foods, such as TV dinners
• preserved meat (such as hot dogs) and luncheon meats
• cheeses of all kinds (including cottage)
• anything preserved in brine, such as olives, pickles, and sauerkraut.

In addition, a patient watching calories should *avoid:*
• sugar and sweets
• high cholesterol foods
• milk, milk products, and coconut oil
• alcoholic beverages

His diet should *include* the following foods, low in sodium:

Fruits and their juices

apples	apricots
bananas	dates
grapefruit	nectarines
oranges	prunes
raisins	watermelon

Vegetables (fresh or frozen)

asparagus	beans
brussels sprouts	cabbage
cauliflower	corn
lima beans	peas
peppers	potatoes
radishes	squash

Cardiac Rehabilitation Plan for Graduated Activity and Exercise

IN HOSPITAL	EXERCISE	ACTIVITY
Day 2	Passive range of motion (ROM) to all extremities in bed; active plantar extension and dorsiflexion	Bedside commode; feed self; groom self
Days 3 and 4	Active ROM (up to 10X)	Bathe self under supervision
Days 5 to 7	Minimal resistance to active ROM 10X each	Walk back and forth in room twice q.i.d.
Days 8 and 9	Moderate resistance to active ROM 10X each	Stand at sink to shave; walk to bathroom
Day 10	Add: Three arm and shoulder motions, five lateral bends and knee raises, and five side leg raises	Take a shower; walk in hall b.i.d.
Days 11 and 12	Add: Sitting on flat bed, touch toes and twist trunk twice	Sit up most of day; walk length of hall b.i.d.
Days 13 and 14	Add: Three standing half-knee bends	Walk at will, including up and down one flight of stairs.

The above regimen is done under the direct supervision of the cardiac rehabilitation team. The activities should terminate whenever the pulse rate exceeds 115 beats/minute, ectopic beats occur, or the patient experiences chest pain.

REHABILITATION

INDEX

INDEX

INDEX

INDEX

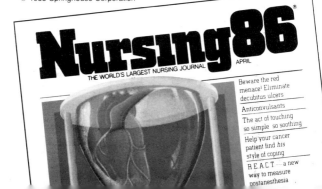